AF823735

Dermatology

An International Journal founded as
'Dermatologische Zeitschrift' by Oskar Lassar (1893–1907)
Continued by Erich Hoffmann (1908–1938), continued as 'Dermatologica' (1939–1991),
by Wilhelm Lutz (1939–1958), Rudolf Schuppli (1959–1985) and J.-H. Saurat (1986–2015),
continued as 'Dermatology' since 1992

Editor-in-Chief

Gregor B.E. Jemec – *University Hospital of Roskilde,* Roskilde, Denmark

Section Editor 'International Dermatology Outcome Measures'

Amit Garg – *Hofstra Northwell School of Medicine,* Hempstead, USA

Section Editor 'Skin Cancer'

Claas Ulrich – *Charité – University Medicine Berlin,* Berlin, Germany

Section Editors 'Tattoo and Body Art'

Nicolas Kluger – *University of Helsinki Central Hospital,* Helsinki, Finland
Jørgen Serup – *Bispebjerg University Hospital,* Copenhagen, Denmark

Associate Editors

Giuseppe Argenziano – *Second University of Naples,* Naples, Italy
Perla Calderón – *University of Chile,* Santiago, Chile
Lars E. French – *University Hospital Zurich,* Zurich, Switzerland
Robert Gniadecki – *Bispebjerg University Hospital,* Copenhagen, Denmark
Qiang Ju – *Renji Hospital, Shanghai Jiao Tong University,* Shanghai, China
Brian Kirby – *St. Vincent's University Hospital,* Dublin, Ireland
Dan Lipsker – *University of Strasbourg,* Strasbourg, France
Branka Marinović – *University Hospital Center Zagreb,* Zagreb, Croatia
Tetsuo Shiohara – *Kyorin University,* Tokyo, Japan
H. Peter Soyer – *The University of Queensland,* Woolloongabba, Australia
Dae Hun Suh – *Seoul National University,* Seoul, Republic of Korea
Jacek C. Szepietowski – *University of Wroclaw,* Wroclaw, Poland
Christos C. Zouboulis – *Dessau City Clinic,* Dessau, Germany

(Continued on next page)

Official Organ of

Swiss Society for Dermatology and Venereology
Schweizerische Gesellschaft für Dermatologie und Venerologie
Société Suisse de Dermatologie et Vénéréologie
sgdv ssdv

Japanese Society for Dermatoallergology and Contact Dermatitis

ESTP research
European Society of Tattoo and Pigment Research

KARGER

Printed in Germany on acid-free and non-aging paper (ISO 9706) by Stückle Druck, Ettenheim

Dermatology

Editorial Board

Tove Agner – *Bispebjerg University Hospital,* Copenhagen, Denmark
Hervé Bachelez – *St. Louis Hospital,* Paris, France
Tania Cestari – *Federal University of Rio Grande do Sul,* Porto Alegre, Brazil
Veronique del Marmol – *Université Libre de Bruxelles,* Brussels, Belgium
Lennart Emtestam – *Karolinska University Hospital and Institutet,* Stockholm, Sweden
Alice Gottlieb – *Tufts University,* Boston, USA
Dimitrios Ioannides – *Aristotle University Medical School,* Thessaloniki, Greece
Marcel F. Jonkman – *University Medical Center Groningen,* Groningen, The Netherlands
Sirkku Peltonen – *University of Turku and Turku University Hospital,* Turku, Finland
Errol P. Prens – *Erasmus Medical Center,* Rotterdam, Netherlands
Luis Puig – *Autonomous University of Barcelona,* Barcelona, Spain
Jean Revuz – *Private Practice – Dermatology,* Paris, France
Eggert Stockfleth – *Ruhr University Bochum,* Bochum, Germany
Devinder Mohan Thappa – *Jawaharlal Institute of Postgraduate Medical Education and Research,* Puducherry, India

KARGER

E-Mail karger@karger.com
www.karger.com

© 2016 S. Karger AG, Basel

The Journal Home Page is available at:
www.karger.com/drm

Dermatology

Guidelines for Authors

Submission
Only original papers written in English should be sent to:

www.karger.com/drm

S. Karger AG
Prof. Dr. Gregor B.E. Jemec
Editorial Office 'Dermatology'
PO Box
CH–4009 Basel (Switzerland)
Tel. +41 61 306 1358
Fax +41 61 306 1434
E-Mail drm@karger.com

Conditions
All manuscripts are subject to editorial review. Manuscripts are received with the explicit understanding that they are not under simultaneous consideration by any other publisher. Submission of an article for publication implies transfer of the copyright from the author to the publisher upon acceptance. Accepted papers become the permanent property of *Dermatology* and may not be reproduced by any means, in whole or in part, without the written consent of the publisher. It is the author's responsibility to obtain permission to reproduce illustrations, tables, etc. from other publications.

Peer Review Policy
Dermatology is a peer-reviewed journal. Our aim is to provide authors with fast and constructive feedback regarding their submitted manuscript. The Editor-in-Chief and international editorial board ensure a thorough and fair peer review and the highest scientific publishing standards. The Editor-in-Chief is responsible for maintaining a high-quality peer review of papers submitted to the journal.

Types of Papers
The journal accepts the following types of papers:

- Original Papers
- Review Papers
- Industry News
- Basic Science Investigations
- Clinical Investigations
- Novel Treatments
- Surgical Pearls
- Consensus Guidelines

Original Papers: Fully documented reports of original research. They must describe full sets of significant, original experiments in basic science and translational research in dermatology. Consideration for publication is based on originality, novelty, scientific soundness and appropriate analysis. An Abstract, Introduction, Materials and Methods, Results and Discussion sections are required. The abstract should be structured and contain the following parts: Background, Objective, Methods, Results, Conclusion; it should have no more than 250 words. A synopsis of the Material and Methods section must be provided in a flow chart. The detailed paragraph will be published as supplementary material. The submission of raw data as supplementary material is strongly encouraged.

Review Papers: Comprehensive reviews covering a timely topic by experts in the field.
Review Papers are usually invited by the Editor but may be unsolicited. An abstract (not structured) of no more than 250 words is required. Review Papers are not subject to page charges, and color illustrations are reproduced free of charge in the printed edition. All published Review Papers are freely accessible online.

Surgical Pearls: Presentation of novel surgical techniques and discussion of their advantages compared to current approaches. Papers of this type should include a short video sequence to be published online.

Consensus Guidelines: Consensus guidelines are welcome from societies or working groups to provide guidance in key and emerging areas in all fields of dermatology.

Sections
International Dermatology Outcome Measures: The section includes papers, the research focus of which is in alignment with the mission of the non-profit organization 'International Dermatology Outcome Measures' (IDEOM): The development of evidence-based outcomes measures to evaluate the impact of treatments for patients with dermatological diseases. Please view the above 'Types of Papers' list for all different paper categories accepted within this section. All submissions to this section are subject to editorial and peer-review. *Dermatology* publication conditions apply.

Skin Cancer: The section with a thematic focus on Skin Cancer includes papers on any cancers that arise from the skin (basal-cell cancer (BCC), squamous-cell cancer (SCC) and melanoma). Please view the above 'Types of Papers' list for all different paper categories accepted within this section. All submissions to this section are subject to editorial and peer-review. *Dermatology* publication conditions apply.

Tattoo and Body Art: Dermatology welcomes submissions to the section 'Tattoo and Body Art' covering various types of body art and skin modifications (namely tattooing, permanent make-up, body-piercing, scarification, etc.) and including basic research and science on those topics. Please view the above 'Types of Papers' list for all paper categories accepted within this section. All submissions to this section are subject to editorial and peer-review. *Dermatology* publication conditions apply.

Ethics
Published research must comply with the guidelines for human studies and animal welfare regulations. Authors should state that subjects have given their informed consent and that the study protocol has been approved by the institute's committee on human research. Further, they should also state that animal experiments conform to institutional standards.

Conflicts of Interest
Authors are required to disclose any sponsorship or funding arrangements relating to their research, and all authors should disclose any possible conflicts of interest. Conflict of interest statements will be published at the end of the article.

Plagiarism Policy
Whether intentional or not, plagiarism is a serious violation. We define plagiarism as a case in which a paper reproduces another work with at least 25% similarity and without citation. If evidence of plagiarism is found before/after acceptance or after publication of the paper, the author will be offered a chance for rebuttal. If the arguments are not found to be satisfactory, the manuscript will be retracted and the author sanctioned from publishing papers for a period to be determined by the responsible Editor.

Arrangement
Papers should comprise approximately 13 double-spaced manuscript pages including figures, tables and references. For technical details please refer to: **www.karger.com/electronic_submission**.

Title page: The first page of each paper should indicate the title, the authors' names, the institute where the work was conducted and a short title for use as running head.

Full address: The exact postal address of the corresponding author complete with postal code must be given at the bottom of the title page. Please also supply phone and fax numbers, as well as e-mail address.

Key words: For indexing purposes, a list of 3–10 key words in English is essential for all papers.

Key message: Kindly provide a sentence of up to 15 words that capture the essence of the content of the paper.

Material and Methods: A synopsis of the Material and Methods section must be provided in a flow chart. The detailed paragraph will be published as supplementary material.

Footnotes: Avoid footnotes. When essential, they are numbered consecutively and typed at the foot of the appropriate page.

Tables and illustrations: Tables and illustrations (both numbered in Arabic numerals) should be stored in separate files. Tables require a heading and figures a legend, also prepared in a separate file. When possible, group several illustrations in one block for reproduction (max. size 180 × 223 mm) or provide crop marks. B/w half-tone and color illustrations must have a final resolution of 300 dpi after scaling, line drawings one of 800–1,200 dpi. For further details, please refer to the Submission Website at **www.karger.com/drm**.

Color illustrations: All color illustrations will be published in color online and black/white in print. In print, optional publication of illustrations in color is subject to a charge of CHF 250.00 per page.

KARGER
E-Mail karger@karger.com
www.karger.com
© 2016 S. Karger AG, Basel
The Guidelines for Authors are available at:
www.karger.com/drm_Guidelines

No charges are imposed for color illustrations of Review Papers.

References: In the text identify references by Arabic numerals [in square brackets]. Material submitted for publication but not yet accepted should be noted as [unpublished data] and not be included in the reference list. The list of references should include only those publications which are cited in the text. Avoid using abstracts and posters as references. If necessary, list as footnotes in standard reference format, followed by the designation '(abstr.)' or '(poster)'. For posters, add the details of the meeting where presented.
Do not alphabetize; number references in the order in which they are first mentioned in the text. The surnames of the authors followed by initials should be given. There should be no punctuation other than a comma to separate the authors. Preferably, please cite all authors. Abbreviate journal names according to the Index Medicus system. Also see International Committee of Medical Journal Editors: Uniform requirements for manuscripts submitted to biomedical journals (www.icmje.org).

Examples
(a) Papers published in periodicals: Chatel JM, Bernard H, Orson FM: Isolation and characterization of two complete Ara h 2 isoforms cDNA. Int Arch Allergy Immunol 2003;131:14–18.
(b) Papers published only with DOI numbers: Theoharides TC, Boucher W, Spear K: Serum interleukin-6 reflects disease severity and osteoporosis in mastocytosis patients. Int Arch Allergy Immunol DOI: 10.1159/000063858.
(c) Monographs: Matthews DE, Farewell VT: Using and Understanding Medical Statistics, ed 3, revised. Basel, Karger, 1996.
(d) Edited books: DuBois RN: Cyclooxygenase-2 and colorectal cancer; in Dannenberg AJ, Dubois RN (eds): COX-2. Prog Exp Tum Res. Basel, Karger, 2003, vol 37, pp 124–137.

Reference Management Software: Use of EndNote is recommended for easy management and formatting of citations and reference lists.

Digital Object Identifier (DOI)
S. Karger Publishers supports DOIs as unique identifiers for articles. A DOI number will be printed on the title page of each article. DOIs can be useful in the future for identifying and citing articles published online without volume or issue information. More information can be found at **www.doi.org**.

Supplementary Material
Multimedia files and other supplementary files, directly relevant but not essential to the conclusions of a paper, enhance the online version of a publication and increase its visibility on the web. These files will undergo editorial review. The Editors reserve the right to limit the scope and length of the supplementary material. Multimedia and supplementary material should meet production quality standards for publication without the need for any modification or editing. Files should not exceed 10 MB in size. Figures and tables need to have titles and legends, and all files should be supplied separately and labeled clearly. All supplementary material should be referred to in the main text. A DOI number will be assigned to supplementary material and it will be hosted online at https://karger.figshare.com under a CC BY license. Authors will be charged a processing fee of CHF 250.00 for supplementary material.

Self-Archiving/Green Open Access
Karger permits authors to archive their pre-prints (i.e. pre-peer review) or post-prints (i.e. accepted manuscript after peer review but before production) on their personal or their institution's internal website. In addition, authors may post their accepted manuscripts in public Open Access repositories and scientific networks (e.g. ResearchGate or Mendeley) no earlier than 12 months following publication of the final version of their article. For all self-archiving, the posted manuscripts must:

- Be used for noncommercial purposes only
- Be linked to the final version on www.karger.com
- Include the following statement:

'This is the peer-reviewed but unedited manuscript version of the following article: [insert full citation, e.g. Cytogenet Genome Res 2014;142:227–238 (DOI: 10.1159/000361001)]. The final, published version is available at http://www.karger.com/?doi=[insert DOI number].'

It is the author's responsibility to fulfill these requirements.

For papers published online first with a DOI number only, full citation details must be added as soon as the paper is published in its final version. This is important to ensure that citations can be credited to the article.
Manuscripts to be archived in PubMed Central due to funding requirements will be submitted by Karger on the author's behalf [see Funding Organizations (NIH etc.)].

For self-archiving Author's Choice™ (Gold Open Access) articles, see Author's Choice™.

Author's Choice™
Karger's Author's Choice™ service broadens the reach of your article and gives all users worldwide free and full access for reading, downloading and printing at www.karger.com. The option is available for a one-time fee of CHF 3,000.00, which is a permissible cost in grant allocation. More information can be found at www.karger.com/authors_choice.
The final, published version of the article may be posted at any time and in any repository or on other websites, in accordance with the relevant Creative Commons license. Reposted Open Access articles must:

- Follow the terms of the relevant Creative Commons license
- Be linked to the final version on www.karger.com
- Include the following statement:

'The final, published version of this article is available at http://www.karger.com/?doi=[insert DOI number].'

It is the author's responsibility to fulfill these requirements.

For papers published online first with a DOI number only, full citation details must be added as soon as the paper is published in its final version. This is important to ensure that citations can be credited to the article.

Funding Organizations (NIH etc.)
The U.S. National Institutes of Health (NIH) Public Access Policy mandates that accepted, peer-reviewed manuscripts are archived in its digital database, PubMed Central (PMC), within 12 months of the official publication date. As a service to authors, Karger submits NIH-funded articles to PMC on behalf of the authors immediately upon publication. The NIH assigns a PMCID within approximately 1 month and the manuscript will appear in PMC after a 12-month embargo. For authors making their paper Open Access through Author's Choice™, the embargo will be overridden, thereby accelerating the accessibility of the article. Karger also complies with other funders' requirements (including Wellcome Trust and RCUK) for submission to PMC. Authors should include information on their grants in the Acknowledgements section of their papers.

Page Charges
There are no page charges for papers of 4 or fewer printed pages (including tables, illustrations and references). Each additional complete or partial page is charged to the author at CHF 325.00. The allotted size of a paper is equal to approximately 13 double-spaced manuscript pages (including tables, illustrations and references).

Proofs
Unless indicated otherwise, proofs are sent to the corresponding author and should be returned with the least possible delay. Alterations other than the correction of printer's errors are charged to the author.

E-Pub First
All articles are published electronically ahead of print with a DOI number and are supplemented later with the definite reference of the printed version. The articles become available immediately after the authors' approval to publication, with the added advantage of being citable much earlier than in print. Authors can influence the time of appearance by promptly returning the proofs.

Reprints
Order forms are sent with the proofs. Orders submitted after the issue has been printed are subject to considerably higher prices.

KARGER
E-Mail karger@karger.com
www.karger.com

© 2016 S. Karger AG, Basel

The Guidelines for Authors are available at:
www.karger.com/drm_Guidelines

Dermatology

General Information

ISSN Print Edition: 1018–8665
ISSN Online Edition: 1421–9832

Journal Homepage: www.karger.com/drm

Publication Data: *Dermatology* is published 6 times a year. Volume 232 with 6 issues appears in 2016.

Copyright: © 2016 S. Karger AG, Basel (Switzerland). All rights reserved. No part of this publication may be translated into other languages, reproduced or utilized in any form or by any means, electronic or mechanical, including photocopying, recording, microcopying, or by any information storage and retrieval system, without permission in writing from the publisher or, in the case of photocopying, direct payment of a specified fee to the Copyright Clearance Center.

Disclaimer: The statements, opinions and data contained in this publication are solely those of the individual authors and contributors and not of the publisher and the editor(s). The appearance of advertisements in the journal is not a warranty, endorsement, or approval of the products or services advertised or of their effectiveness, quality or safety. The publisher and the editor(s) disclaim responsibility for any injury to persons or property resulting from any ideas, methods, instructions or products referred to in the content or advertisements.

Subscription Rates: Subscriptions run for a full calendar year. Prices are given per year.

Personal subscription:

Print or Online	**Print+Online combined**
CHF 1579.00	CHF 1629.00
EUR 1410.00	EUR 1450.00
USD 1698.00	USD 1752.00

postage and handling (added to print and print+online)
CHF 45.60 Europe, CHF 67.20 Overseas
EUR 40.80
USD 62.40

Institutional subscription:

Print or Online	**Print+Online combined**
CHF 3157.00	CHF 3631.00
EUR 2819.00	EUR 3242.00
USD 3395.00	USD 3904.00

postage and handling (added to print and print+online)
CHF 57.00 Europe, CHF 84.00 Overseas
EUR 51.00
USD 78.00

Discount subscription prices:
For members of Dermatology Societies.

Back Volumes and Single Issues: Information on availability and prices of single print issues and print or electronic back volumes can be obtained from Customer Service at *service@karger.com.*

Bibliographic Indices: This journal is regularly listed in bibliographic services, including *Current Contents*® and PubMed/MEDLINE.

Photocopying: This journal has been registered with the Copyright Clearance Center (CCC), as indicated by the code appearing on the first page of each article. For readers in the US, this code signals consent for copying of articles for personal or internal use, or for the personal or internal use of specific clients, provided that the stated fee is paid per copy directly to
Copyright Clearance Center Inc.
222 Rosewood Drive
Danvers, MA 01923 (USA)
A copy of the first page of the article must accompany payment. Consent does not extend to copying for general distribution, for promotion, for creating new works, or for resale. In these cases, specific written permission must be obtained from the copyright owner,
S. Karger AG, P.O. Box
CH–4009 Basel (Switzerland).

Subscription Orders:
Orders can be placed at agencies, bookstores, directly with the Publisher

S. Karger AG
Medical and Scientific Publishers
Allschwilerstrasse 10
CH–4009 Basel
Switzerland

t: +41 61 306 11 11
f: +41 61 306 12 34
e: karger@karger.com
w: www.karger.com

(for courier services only:
Allschwilerstrasse 10
CH–4055 Basel)

or further Karger offices
or representatives:

Germany
S. Karger GmbH
Postfach
79095 Freiburg
Deutschland
(Hausadresse: Wilhelmstrasse 20A,
79098 Freiburg)
t: +49 761 45 20 70
f: +49 761 45 20 714
e: information@karger.de
w: www.karger.de

Japan
Karger Japan, Inc.
Shiba Daimon Asahi Bldg. 2F
1-2-23 Shiba Daimon
Minato-ku
Tokyo 105-0012
Japan
t: +81 3 6435 6242
f: +81 3 6435 6244
e: publisher@karger.jp
w: www.karger.jp

USA
S. Karger Publishers, Inc.
26 West Avon Road
P.O. Box 529
Unionville, CT 06085
USA
Toll free: +1 800 828 5479
t: +1 860 675 7834
f: +1 860 675 7302
e: kargerusa@karger.com

France
Enter & Read
Albertine Luginbuhl
23, rue du Départ, boite 37
75014 Paris
France
t: +33 (0) 6 81 04 76 85
e: albertineluginbuhl@orange.fr

South East Asia, China and Taiwan
Karger Regional Office (Malaysia)
Level 28-03-03A, PJ Exchange
No. 16A, Persiaran Barat
46050 Petaling Jaya
Selangor Darul Ehsan
Malaysia
t: +60 3 7962 0158
f: +60 3 7962 0001
e: service@karger.cn; r.chew@karger.cn

Karger China
51F Raffles City Centre
268 Xi Zang Middle Road
Huang Pu District
Shanghai 200001
P.R. China
t: +86 21 2312 7673
f: +86 21 2312 7777
e: service@karger.cn
r.chew@karger.cn
w: www.karger.cn

India, Bangladesh, Sri Lanka
Karger India
Plot No. 17, Yusuf Sarai Market
B.L. Glass Building, 2nd Floor
Sri Aurobindo Marg
New Delhi 110 016
India
t: +91 11 46029 633
f: +91 11 46029 634
c: +91 98 91052 128
e: r.kumar@kargerindia.com
w: www.karger.com

Change of Address:
Both old and new address should be sent to the subscription source.

KARGER

© 2016 S. Karger AG, Basel

E-Mail karger@karger.com
www.karger.com

The Journal Home Page is available at:
www.karger.com/drm

Medical Statistics has never been easier!

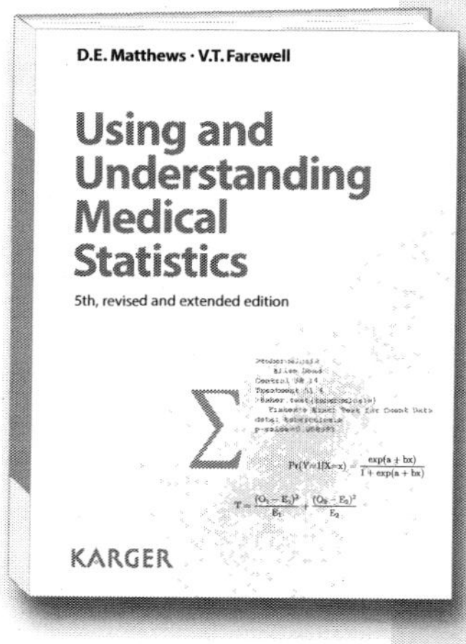

David E. Matthews
Vernon T. Farewell

Using and Understanding Medical Statistics

5th, revised and extended edition

Matthews, D.E. (Waterloo, Ont.);
Farewell, V.T. (Cambridge)
Using and Understanding Medical Statistics
5th, revised and extended edition
XX + 338 p., 48 fig., 103 tab., 2015
CHF 49.00 / EUR 46.00 / USD 54.00
(hard cover + online supplementary material)
Online version for institutional purchase
Prices subject to change, VAT not included
EUR price for eurozone countries, USD price for USA and Latin America only
ISBN 978-3-318-05458-3
(hard cover + online supplementary material)
e-ISBN 978-3-318-05459-0

eBook available on:

Google play amazon
Vitalsource

Dear Librarian

I have reviewed this publication and would like to recommend it for our library.

Recommended by:

Department:

Date:

Signature:

Orders may be placed with any bookshop, subscription agency, directly with the publisher or through a Karger distributor.

The fifth revised edition of this highly successful book presents the most extensive enhancement since *Using and Understanding Medical Statistics* was first published 30 years ago. Without question, the single greatest change has been the inclusion of source code, together with selected output, for the award-winning, open-source, statistical package known as R. This innovation has enabled the authors to de-emphasize formulae and calculations, and let software do all of the 'heavy lifting'.
This edition also introduces readers to several graphical statistical tools, such as Q-Q plots to check normality, residual plots for multiple regression models, funnel plots to detect publication bias in a meta-analysis and Bland-Altman plots for assessing agreement in clinical measurements. New examples that better serve the expository goals have been added to a half-dozen chapters. In addition, there are new sections describing exact confidence bands for the Kaplan-Meier estimator, as well as negative binomial and zero-inflated Poisson regression models for over-dispersed count data.
The end result is not only an excellent introduction to medical statistics, but also an invaluable reference for every discerning reader of medical research literature.

Contents

Preface to the Fifth Edition
Prefaces to the Previous Editions

- Basic Concepts
- Tests of Significance
- Fisher's Test for 2×2 Contingency Tables
- Approximate Significance Tests for Contingency Tables
- Some Warnings concerning 2×2 Tables
- Kaplan-Meier or 'Actuarial' Survival Curves
- The Log-Rank or Mantel-Haenszel Test for Comparing Survival Curves
- An Introduction to the Normal Distribution
- Analyzing Normally Distributed Data
- Linear Regression Models for Medical Data
- Binary Logistic Regression
- Regression Models for Count Data
- Proportional Hazards Regression
- The Analysis of Longitudinal Data
- Analysis of Variance
- Data Analysis
- The Question of Sample Size
- The Design of Clinical Trials
- Further Comments regarding Clinical Trials
- Meta-Analysis
- Epidemiological Applications
- Diagnostic Tests
- Agreement and Reliability

References
Subject Index

The easiest way to order: **www.karger.com/medical_statistics**

Karger – Medical and Scientific Publishers
CH–4009 Basel, Switzerland
orders@karger.com, f: +41 61 306 12 34
www.karger.com

KI15406

KARGER 125 YEARS

Dermatology

Therapeutic Use of Ingenol Mebutate in Dermatology

Guest Editor
Günther F.L. Hofbauer, Zurich

27 figures in color, 2016

KARGER Basel · Freiburg · Paris · London · New York · Chennai · New Delhi · Bangkok · Beijing · Shanghai · Tokyo · Kuala Lumpur · Singapore · Sydney

Disclosure Statement Guest Editor

Research support was given by Almirall, Biofrontera, Clinuvel, Galderma Spirig, LEO Pharma, L'Oréal, MEDA, La Roche-Posay, Sunlight Research Forum, Wyeth/Pfizer, and Vivosight.

Speaker's fees were paid by AbbVie, Galderma Spirig, LEO Pharma, L'Oréal, MEDA, MedUpdate, Merck, Novartis, Pierre Fabre, and Pfizer.

Consulting was provided to AbbVie, Biofrontera/Louis Widmer, Galderma Spirig, Hoffmann-La Roche, LEO Pharma, and MEDA.

This publication was sponsored by LEO Pharma.
http://www.leo-pharma.ch/

S. Karger
Medical and Scientific Publishers
Basel · Freiburg · Paris · London · New York · Chennai · New Delhi · Bangkok · Beijing · Shanghai · Tokyo · Kuala Lumpur · Singapore · Sydney

Disclaimer
The statements, opinions and data contained in this publication are solely those of the individual authors and contributors and not of the publisher and the editor(s). The appearance of advertisements in the journal is not a warranty, endorsement, or approval of the products or services advertised or of their effectiveness, quality or safety. The publisher and the editor(s) disclaim responsibility for any injury to persons or property resulting from any ideas, methods, instructions or products referred to in the content or advertisements.

Drug Dosage
The authors and the publisher have exerted every effort to ensure that drug selection and dosage set forth in this text are in accord with current recommendations and practice at the time of publication. However, in view of ongoing research, changes in government regulations, and the constant flow of information relating to drug therapy and drug reactions, the reader is urged to check the package insert for each drug for any change in indications and dosage and for added warnings and precautions. This is particularly important when the recommended agent is a new and/or infrequently employed drug.

All rights reserved.
No part of this publication may be translated into other languages, reproduced or utilized in any form or by any means, electronic or mechanical, including photocopying, recording, microcopying, or by any information storage and retrieval system, without permission in writing from the publisher or, in the case of photocopying, direct payment of a specified fee to the Copyright Clearance Center (see 'General Information').

© Copyright 2016 by S. Karger AG, Basel
P.O. Box, CH–4009 Basel (Switzerland)
ISBN 978–3–318–05909–0
e-ISBN 978–3–318–05910–6

KARGER

E-Mail karger@karger.com
www.karger.com/drm

Vol. 232, Suppl. 1, 2016

Dermatology

Contents

© 2016 S. Karger AG, Basel

E-Mail karger@karger.com
www.karger.com/drm

Dermatology

Dermatology 2016;232(suppl 1):IV
DOI: 10.1159/000447385

Published online: August 11, 2016

Preface

Dermatology is an experimenting discipline. While new treatments for specific diseases keep getting registered, we still have a shortage of treatments for many skin conditions. It is thus rather the rule than the exception to adopt treatment strategies available to unregistered indications as off-label use in our specialty. Dermatologists also excel in personalizing medicine for their patients by adapting registered treatment protocols to fit their patient needs while achieving clinical improvement.

Here, we present to you a collection of cases in which the substance ingenol mebutate that was recently registered for the treatment of actinic keratosis is put to use with regimens deviating from the registered ones and also beyond the realm of actinic keratoses. The authors have varied their application schemes to accommodate for larger treatment fields, the use of ingenol mebutate with occlusion and with a reduced number of applications to treat actinic keratoses. Other cases illustrate the authors' experience in conditions beyond actinic keratoses such as Bowen's disease, warts, basal cell carcinoma and lentigo maligna. While a case report does not prove efficacy on its own, case reporting is an important first step in the discovery of new uses and treatment regimens for ingenol mebutate. We hope to inspire the readers with our collection of cases to do what dermatologists do best – personalize medicine for our patients.

Günther F.L. Hofbauer, Zurich

KARGER

© 2016 S. Karger AG, Basel

1018–8665/16/2327–00IV$39.50/0

E-Mail karger@karger.com
www.karger.com/drm

Dermatology

Dermatology 2016;232(suppl 1):1–3
DOI: 10.1159/000447386

Published online: August 11, 2016

Ingenol Mebutate for Recalcitrant Chronic Actinic Cheilitis

Evangelia Tzika Isabelle Masouyé Michael Mühlstädt Emmanuel Laffitte

Division of Dermatology and Venereology, Geneva University Hospitals, Geneva, Switzerland

Key Words
Ingenol mebutate · Chronic actinic cheilitis · Imiquimod · Photodynamic therapy

Abstract
We present the case of a healthy 76-year-old man with a whitish, hyperkeratotic lesion of the lower lip diagnosed as actinic cheilitis (AC) previously treated with classic red light photodynamic therapy 5 years ago. Initial treatment with 5% imiquimod cream – also with intensified application – failed. After 2 cycles thrice daily, consecutive applications of 150 μg/g ingenol mebutate gel at 3 weeks' interval, the lesions cleared completely. Surprisingly, no pustular or crusting reaction or other side effect occurred contrary to expectation. Remission was stable for 10 months, when recurrence occurred. Ingenol mebutate proved to be a feasible and safe treatment in this otherwise refractory case of AC.
© 2016 S. Karger AG, Basel

Introduction

Actinic cheilitis (AC) is an intraepithelial squamous cell carcinoma of the vermilion of the lower lip, caused by chronic continuous damage by ultraviolet light. It is characterized by scaling and crusting of the vermilion of the lip and by a loss of the usually accurate delineation between the vermilion border and the cornified epidermis of the lip. We report a case of AC resistant to treatment with 5% imiquimod cream, successfully treated with 150 μg/g ingenol mebutate gel.

Case Report

A healthy 76-year-old man presented to our clinic with a whitish, hyperkeratotic lesion of the lower lip (fig. 1). He reported previous treatment with classic, red light photodynamic therapy by his dermatologist 5 years ago with little benefit. The clinical diagnosis of AC was confirmed by skin biopsy showing epithelial atrophy and a moderate dermal actinic elastosis, compatible with AC. The patient did not have any known history of labial herpes and had reported no bouts of this disease with previous photodynamic treatment; so we deemed prophylactic treatment with an anti-herpetic agent such as valaciclovir unnecessary. This should, however, always be evaluated and decided individually in every patient. Initial treatment consisted of topical 5% imiquimod cream thrice a week. Only insufficient inflammation was evoked after 6 applications without clinical improvement; thus, the frequency of application was increased to once daily for 1 month (fig. 2). Again, insufficient inflammation was evoked without clinical improvement. The patient then received a first treatment cycle of 150 μg/g ingenol mebutate gel once daily for 3 consecutive days, an off-label treatment considering the location. Albeit no pustular or crusting reaction – as typically expected with this treatment – occurred but we observed a marked improvement in clinical appearance with reduced scaling of the lower lip. We prescribed an additional cycle of 3 consecutive once-daily applica-

KARGER

E-Mail karger@karger.com
www.karger.com/drm

© 2016 S. Karger AG, Basel
1018–8665/16/2327–0001$39.50/0

Emmanuel Laffitte
Division of Dermatology and Venereology, Geneva University Hospitals
Rue Gabrielle-Perret-Gentil 4
CH–1205 Geneva (Switzerland)
E-Mail ella@hcuge.ch

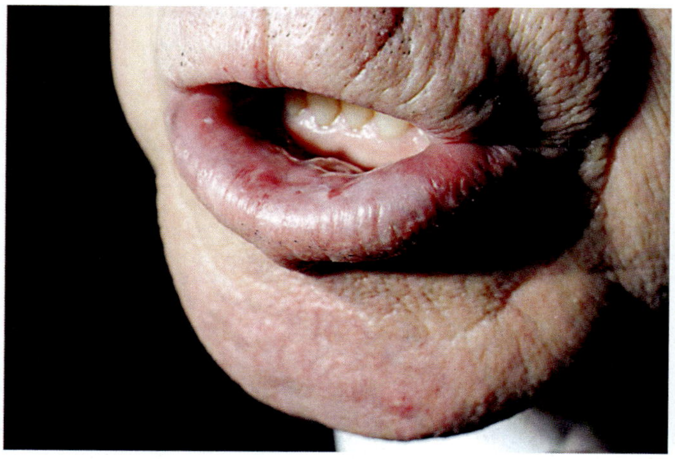

Fig. 1. Before treatment with 5% imiquimod gel.

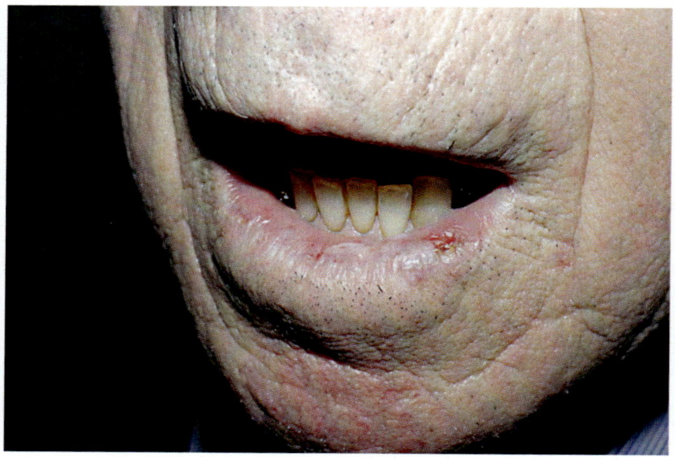

Fig. 2. After treatment with 5% imiquimod gel.

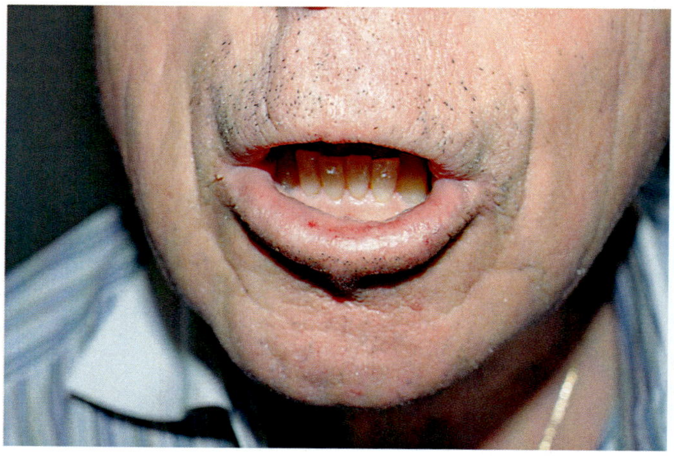

Fig. 3. Three months after treatment with 3 once-daily applications of ingenol mebutate 150 μg/g gel.

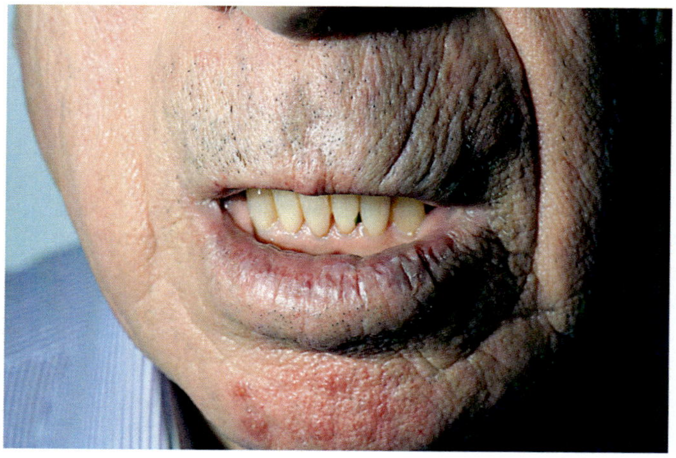

Fig. 4. Recurrence 10 months after treatment with ingenol mebutate 150 μg/g gel once-daily on 3 consecutive days.

tions of 150 μg/g ingenol mebutate gel after 3 weeks for residual lesions (fig. 3). We then noted complete clinical response in absence of any local skin reactions. This remission lasted for about 10 months (fig. 4) until cheilitis reappeared. We treated this with another cycle of 3 once-daily applications of 150 μg/g ingenol mebutate gel, leading to clinical remission once more.

Discussion

AC is a common condition with the potential to progress to invasive squamous cell carcinoma. Treatment modalities comprise classic dermatosurgery (vermilionectomy), cryosurgery, topical 5-fluorouracil, topical imiquimod, conventional and pulsed carbon dioxide lasers, chemical peel, photodynamic therapy and electrodessication with varying cure rates and distinct side effects. Ingenol mebutate is a macrocyclic diterpene ester, registered for the treatment of actinic keratosis [1]. In order to achieve its therapeutic effect, this molecule usually provokes a transitory intense inflammatory reaction including redness and oozing, pustules and crusts on the site of the application. It has been described as a possible therapeutic option in several case reports [2, 3]. In our case of recalcitrant AC, 3 once-daily applications of 150 μg/g ingenol mebutate gel on 3 consecutive days were able to clear the disease without any local skin reaction. This remission lasted for about 10 months, after which a mild cheilitis recurred. The recurrence was again successfully treated with a cycle of ingenol mebutate.

Treatment of AC with 150 μg/g ingenol mebutate gel proved to be a feasible and safe method of treatment in this otherwise refractory case.

Statement of Ethics

Subject has given his informed consent.

Disclosure Statement

Emmanuel Laffitte and Michael Mühlstädt served as speaker and/or advisor for LEO Pharma.

References

1 Fachinformation. Picato® 150 mcg/g, Gel, Picato® 500 mcg/g, Gel. http://www.swissmedicinfo.ch/ShowText.aspx?textType=FI&lang=DE&authNr=62763.

2 Barrado Solís N, Molés Poveda P, Lloret Ruiz C, Pont Sanjuan V, Velasco Pastor M, Quecedo Estébanez E, Miquel Miquel J: Ingenol mebutate gel treatment for actinic cheilitis: report of four cases. Dermatol Ther 2015;28:79–82.

3 Smith KJ, Germain M, Yeager J, Skelton H: Topical 5% imiquimod for the therapy of actinic cheilitis. J Am Acad Dermatol 2002;47:497–501.

Dermatology

Dermatology 2016;232(suppl 1):4–6
DOI: 10.1159/000447387

Published online: August 11, 2016

Ingenol Mebutate 500 μg on the Cheekbones with Concomitant Conjunctivitis

Olivier Gaide   Vincent Cattin

Department of Dermatology and Venerology, CHUV, Lausanne, Switzerland

Key Words
Ingenol mebutate · Conjunctivitis · Cheekbones · Actinic keratosis · Side effects · Healing

Abstract
Ingenol mebutate induces strong inflammation after a single application already. This must be taken into account when prescribing the drug, as mistakes in the application may results in severe side effects. Here, we report the case of a 72-year-old woman who applied ingenol mebutate on the cheekbones and developed a pronounced conjunctivitis, needing topical corticosteroids. The treatment was intended for the actinic keratosis she had on the chest, and the regimen of 2 consecutive once daily applications of ingenol mebutate at 500 μg/g had been prescribed as registered. The inadvertent application on the thin skin of the cheekbones led to a pronounced inflammation. With topical steroids followed by fusidic acid, both conjunctivitis and skin inflammation resolved within a few days. The skin showed erythema for a few weeks, but after 3 months, the patient presented a perfectly smooth skin and was very happy with the cosmetic outcome. This suggests that the cheekbones are a sensitive site for ingenol mebutate, but that intense inflammation should not scare physician or patient, as clinical remission with excellent healing can still be expected.

© 2016 S. Karger AG, Basel

Case Report

A 72-year-old woman consulted our outpatient clinic for small rough skin patches that could be scraped away but typically reappeared after a few months. She was otherwise healthy for her age. Clinical examination revealed numerous actinic keratoses (AKs) of the sun-exposed areas, that is, the back of the hands, the upper chest and the cheekbones. The lesions were too numerous to treat with cryotherapy and clearly constituted field carcinogenesis. We therefore proposed a choice of topical agents for AKs. The patient decided on the simplicity of application of ingenol mebutate and its relatively short treatment and thus total down-time, as she wanted to be able to return to her normal social activities as fast as possible. We initiated ingenol mebutate therapy, starting on the back of the hands and chest using the 500 μg/g regimen, which was to be followed a little later for the face with a lower concentration of 150 μg/g. We obviously failed to sufficiently explain our strategy, as the patient returned the next morning having applied 500 μg/g gel on all areas. The reaction on the hands and chest was normal and evolved as expected, but the local skin reactions on the face were concerning (fig. 1). She presented with swollen eyelids and very pronounced skin inflammation on the cheekbones with erythema and superficial erosion. Her conjunctivae were also involved with pronounced erythema, but without purulent discharge. Burning pain and photophobia were important, associated symptoms. The burning sensation was rated on a Visual Analogue Scale at 7/10. Palpation of the cephalic and cervical lymph nodes was within the norm, with several small LN apparent yet neither swollen nor tender. Our ophthalmologist checked for signs of keratitis and corneal erosions using fluorescein, and neither was present. He initiated corticosteroid eye drops (dexamethasone 0.1%), and we initiated topical corticosteroids and antibiotics (betameth-

KARGER

E-Mail karger@karger.com
www.karger.com/drm

© 2016 S. Karger AG, Basel
1018–8665/16/2327–0004$39.50/0

Olivier Gaide
Service de Dermatologie-Vénéréologie, CHUV
Av. de Beaumont 29
CH–1011 Lausanne (Switzerland)
E-Mail olivier.gaide@chuv.ch

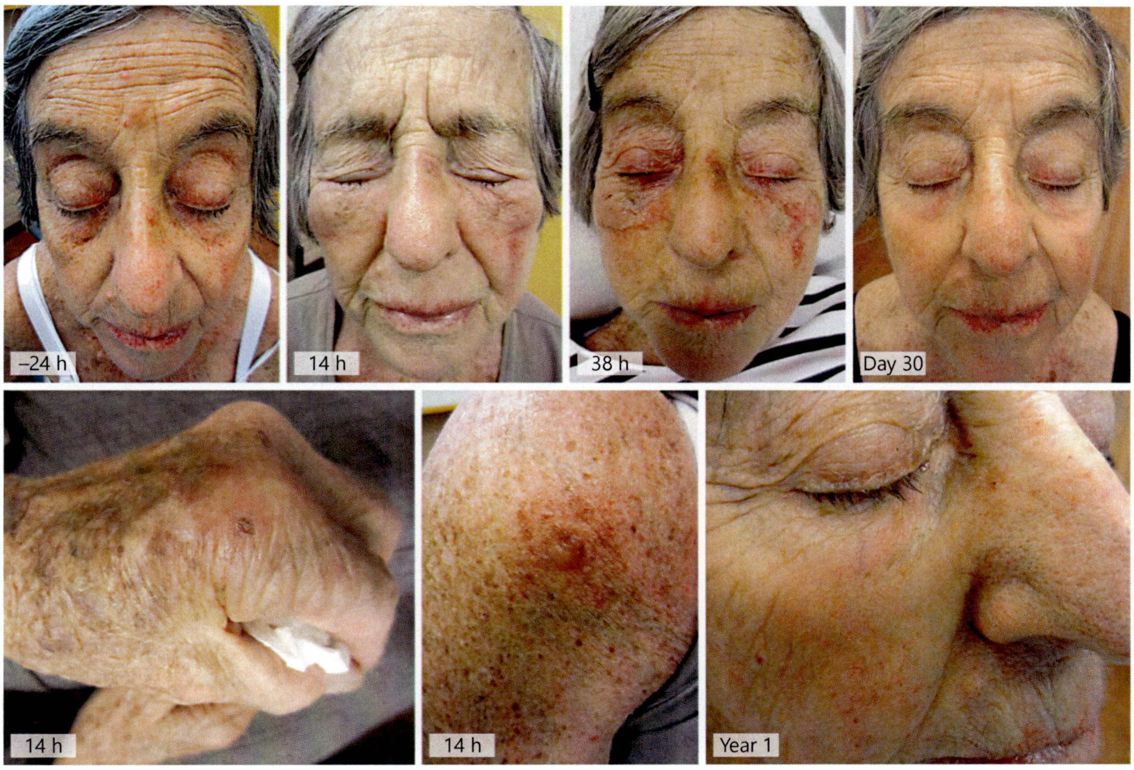

Fig. 1. 24 h before ingenol mebutate, presence of actinic keratosis and solar lentigines. 14 h after a singe application of ingenol mebutate, severe edema and erythema of the cheekbones and eyelids. In comparison, the back of the hand and the shoulder show mild inflammation. 38 h after the single application, edema had subsided, leaving a superficial erosion. 30 days after the application, excellent cosmesis with smooth skin was noted. Year 1, the skin remains devoid of actinic keratosis and lentigines.

asone 0.5% gentamycin 1%) and mefenamic acid (500 mg 3×/j). The clinical course quickly turned positive. After 24 h, edema and conjunctivitis had essentially subsided, and the treatment could be reduced to local fusidic acid for 5 days, as the erosion on the cheekbones was still important. After 10 days, epithelialization was complete, leaving the skin thin and erythematous with a smooth, shiny appearance. Two months later, the skin was looking perfect, with a smoother aspect and the remission of many solar lentigines. This contrasted with the non-treated skin, but the patient was very happy with the rejuvenated aspect of her skin. Two years later, the skin is still looking particularly well, with a rejuvenated look and an absence of any AK recurrences. Hence, the initial, clinically excessive response resulted in a short-term inconvenience and ultimately led to an excellent long-term effect.

Discussion

Although the outcome was very good in the end, a single application of ingenol mebutate 500 µg/g resulted in severe discomfort for the patient. There was no warning sign, no slow start and no possibility to stop the process. This is less likely to happen with an immunomodulator that takes more time to activate inflammation, such as imiquimod. Moreover, imiquimod is acting through plasmacytoid dendritic cells that are infrequent in the normal human conjunctiva and cornea [1]. The risk of triggering inflammation is therefore, at least theoretically, lower. This is in line with our personal experience of imiquimod on the cheekbones or even eyelids, which has not induced such strong reactions in the eye so far in our hands.

The cheekbones are in close proximity to the eyes, and rubbing of the area is a frequent and most often unconscious act. Rubbing can occur in the absence of any eye-itch, especially in the evening when rubbing of the area is thought to decrease eye tension. As a result, drug deposited on the cheekbones can easily be carried toward the eyelids and the eye surface. The temples, the nose and the forehead are all areas of the face where this is less likely to occur. We therefore think that the cheekbones may represent a more risky localization for the use of pro-inflammatory drugs such as ingenol mebutate.

These 2 considerations led us to adapt our clinical practice, and ingenol mebutate is now a second or third choice when treating AKs of the cheekbones.

In conclusion, this case outlines the diversion from prescribed protocol that patients may perform, when the physician has not been careful enough to delineate both what to do and what not to do. Of course, experience teaches one to become better at spotting the possible mishandling of a product. This should not deter the use of ingenol mebutate on the face, which remains a very useful tool in our therapeutic arsenal against AKs. In case of a response judged excessive, topical corticosteroids can be used safely, and without compromising the response to the treatment, as demonstrated by this case, among others [2]. Finally, our case even suggests that the substance offers an interesting tool for skin rejuvenation, as noted by others [3], although this requires further studies to be proven.

Statement of Ethics

Informed consent to use images was provided by the patient.

Disclosure Statement

We have no conflict of interest to declare.

References

1 Chen P, Denniston AK, Hirani S, Hannes S, Nussenblatt RB: Role of dendritic cell subsets in immunity and their contribution to noninfectious uveitis. Surv Ophthalmol 2015;60:242–249.
2 Erlendsson AM, Karmisholt KE, Haak CS, Stender IM, Haedersdal M: Topical corticosteroid has no influence on inflammation or efficacy after ingenol mebutate treatment of grade I to III actinic keratoses (AK): a randomized clinical trial. J Am Acad Dermatol 2016;74:709–715.
3 Braun SA, Gerber PA: Cosmetic effects of ingenol mebutate gel in the treatment of field-cancerized photodamaged skin. Dermatol Surg 2015;41:1328–1329.

Dermatology

Dermatology 2016;232(suppl 1):7–8
DOI: 10.1159/000447388

Published online: August 11, 2016

Ingenol Mebutate 500 μg for Treatment of the Scalp in Refractory Field Cancerization

Olivier Gaide Helena Clayton Marie Girardin Francois Kuonen

Department of Dermatology and Venerology, CHUV, Lausanne, Switzerland

Key Words
Ingenol mebutate · Field cancerization · Immunosuppression · Actinic keratosis · LLC · Scalp

Abstract
Patients suffering from chronic lymphocytic leukemia often develop actinic keratosis (AK) and squamous cell carcinoma in sun-exposed areas. In these particular patients, who have a suboptimal immune function, AK treatment can be particularly challenging. We report the case of a patient who failed to respond to most AK treatments, including 5-FU, imiquimod and photodynamic therapy, but responded to ingenol mebutate. We started with 3 applications of 150 μg/g (registered treatment of the scalp) and also 2 applications of 500 μg/g (registered in for trunk and extremities). Both treatments were well tolerated, but only the latter led to significant clinical success. This suggests that 500 μg/g of ingenol mebutate may represent an interesting therapeutic option in patients with mild immunosuppression.

© 2016 S. Karger AG, Basel

Case Report

The 68-year-old patient had a history of intense sun exposure that lasted most of his adult life. Together with a fair skin, this led to the development of many actinic keratoses (AKs) on the bald part of his scalp, as well as several squamous cell carcinomas and basal cell carcinomas, which were treated by surgery. The AKs had been treated on numerous occasions with cryotherapy. According to the patient, imiquimod had also been tried, but with little significant effect. We were initially surprised by the notion of lack of success of imiquimod. We, therefore, conducted a new set of applications of imiquimod 5%, once daily for 12 days. To our surprise, there was no noticeable erythema or other sign of inflammation, even after 12 days of continuous application. This lack of inflammatory/immune response probably explains the lack of improvement of the AK he had previously observed. Taking a second look at the patient history, with a special accent on his immune function, we realized that the patient had chronic lymphocytic leukemia (CLL). We deduced that this could account for the lack of response to imiquimod, despite reports that this treatment is efficient in immune-deficient patients [1–4].

We decided to try other agents and focused our treatment on 5-FU and classic photodynamic therapy (PDT). Unfortunately, both modalities failed to improve the situation significantly. Daylight PDT and 5-FU failed to induce any observable response, while conventional PDT had to be discontinued early due to intense pain, which may explain why it did not induce a net clinical response either. Looking for new tools to treat this field carcinogenesis, we decided to employ ingenol mebutate. A course of ingenol mebutate as registered with 3 days of daily application of 150 μg/g resulted in a mild inflammation of the treated area (not shown), the first ever observed in this patient. The scalp was smoother after therapy, but 3 months later, the AK count had risen back to the initial level. Since the inflammation had been quite moderate, we switched to 500 μg/g of ingenol mebutate as an off-label treatment, starting on a hemi-scalp. This led to a more robust inflammation at day 4, well within the normal response we routinely observe with the 150 μg/g regimen (fig. 1). The AK response

KARGER

E-Mail karger@karger.com
www.karger.com/drm

© 2016 S. Karger AG, Basel
1018–8665/16/2327–0007$39.50/0

Olivier Gaide
Service de Dermatologie-Vénéréologie, CHUV
Av. de Beaumont 29
CH–1011 Lausanne (Switzerland)
E-Mail olivier.gaide@chuv.ch

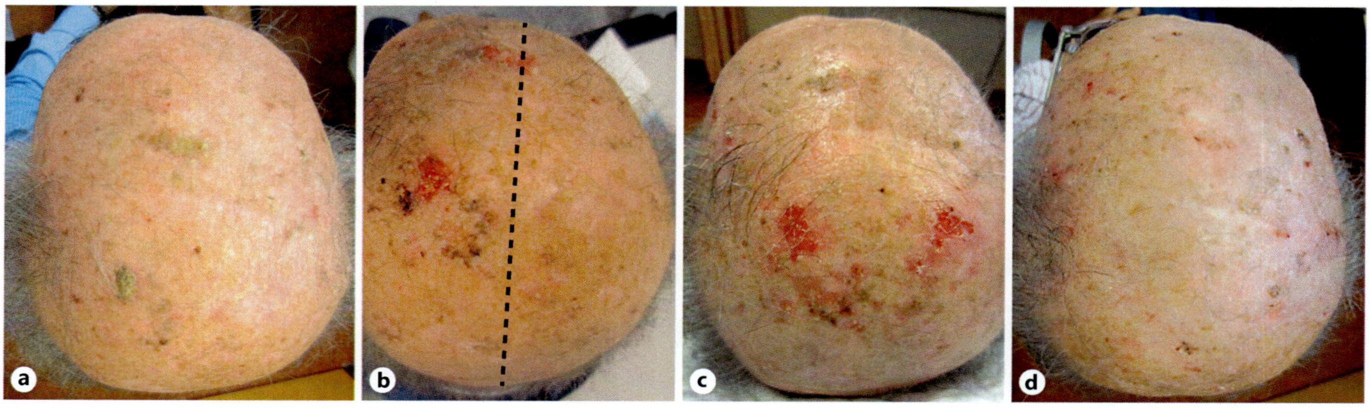

Fig. 1. **a** Initial stage showing numerous AKs. **b** Day 4 after initiation of ingenol mebutate 500 mcg/g on the left side of the scalp. **c** Day 4 after initiation of ingenol mebutate 500 mcg/g on the entire scalp. **d** Skin after 3 cycles of ingenol mebutate 500 and excision of a squamous cell carcinoma of the vertex.

was much better, and using ingenol mebutate 500 at regular intervals of 6 months has allowed us to stabilize the scalp situation, with a net decrease in the number of SCC excision on the scalp.

The CLL slowly worsened during the few past years, prompting our patient's hemato-oncologist to start chemotherapy. The patient has responded well to this therapy, and we now hope that the increased function of his immune system will better keep AKs under control and favor a more prolonged response.

Discussion

In summary, we report the case of a patient responding neither to 5-FU nor imiquimod nor daylight PDT and not tolerating conventional PDT either, but who responded well to a maximized regimen of 500 μg/g ingenol mebutate as an off-label treatment. We think that ingenol mebutate can be a useful option for dermatologists dealing with slightly immune-compromised patients.

Statement of Ethics

Informed consent to use images was provided by the patient.

Disclosure Statement

We have no conflict of interest to declare.

References

1 Perez-Reyes N, Farhi DC: Squamous cell carcinoma of head and neck in patients with well-differentiated lymphocytic lymphoma. Cancer 1987;59:540–544.

2 Levi F, Randimbison L, Te VC, La Vecchia C: Non-hodgkin's lymphomas, chronic lymphocytic leukaemias and skin cancers. Br J Cancer 1996;74:1847–1850.

3 Ulrich C, Bichel J, Euvrard S, Guidi B, Proby CM, van de Kerkhof PC, Amerio P, Rønnevig J, Slade HB, Stockfleth E: Topical immunomodulation under systemic immunosuppression: results of a multicentre, randomized, placebo-controlled safety and efficacy study of imiquimod 5% cream for the treatment of actinic keratoses in kidney, heart, and liver transplant patients. Br J Dermatol 2007;157(suppl 2):25–31.

4 Alessi SS, Sanches JA, Oliveira WR, Messina MC, Pimentel ER, Festa Neto C: Treatment of cutaneous tumors with topical 5% imiquimod cream. Clinics (Sao Paulo) 2009;64:961–966.

Dermatology

Dermatology 2016;232(suppl 1):9–13
DOI: 10.1159/000447389

Published online: August 11, 2016

Successful Treatment of Relapsing Bowen's Disease with Ingenol Mebutate: The Use of Dermoscopy to Monitor the Therapeutic Response

Carlo Mainetti[a] Caroline Guillod[a] Sandra Leoni-Parvex[b]

[a]Department of Dermatology, Ospedale Regionale Bellinzona e Valli, Bellinzona, and [b]Institute of Pathology, Locarno, Switzerland

Key Words

Ingenol mebutate · Bowen's disease · Dermoscopy · Non-melanoma skin cancers

Abstract

Ingenol mebutate (IM) has recently been approved for the topical treatment of actinic keratoses. It appears to have a dual mechanism of action: rapid necrosis after gel application and a subsequent immune-mediated response, which targets any residual dysplastic epidermal cells. We report the successful treatment of a woman, who had been relapsing into Bowen's disease (BD) on her right forefinger for 8 years. During her clinical history, she had received an allogeneic, HLA-identical stem cell transplant for myeloproliferative syndrome with a JAK2V617F mutation and lobectomy of the pulmonary right lower lobe for adenocarcinoma. We used dermoscopy to monitor the therapeutic response of BD. We discuss IM gel as a possible therapeutic option for BD.

© 2016 S. Karger AG, Basel

Introduction

Bowen's disease (BD) is a form of in-situ squamous cell carcinoma (SCC). The typical cutaneous non-pigmented BD presents as a slowly growing, well-demarcated erythematous plaque, with an irregular border and surface scaling or crusting that may erode [1, 2]. Dermoscopy is considered a useful method for the diagnosis of BD based on the typical glomerular vessels plus scaly surface and also for monitoring the therapeutic response of BD [3, 4]. The therapeutic approach for BD includes observation alone and topical and surgical treatments [1, 2].

Ingenol mebutate (IM) is a topical drug recently available for the treatment of actinic keratoses (AK) and was approved in Switzerland in June 2013 for this indication [5]. The advantage of IM compared with other topical agents for AK therapy appears to be its dual mechanism of action – a rapid necrosis after only 2 or 3 days' application of IM gel and the subsequent immune-mediated response – which targets any residual dysplastic epidermal cells [6, 7].

We report the case of a 73-year-old woman with non-pigmented BD on her right forefinger, for which we had tried several local and surgical treatments, which had all led to recurrence of the tumour. A local therapy with IM led to a lasting remission of BD.

Case Report

We report the case of a 73-year-old woman with skin phototype III and with a history of a myeloproliferative syndrome positive for a JAK2V617F mutation and osteomyelofibrosis, which had occurred 17 years ago. She was treated with oral thioguanine and splenectomy at first. Eight years after the initial diagnosis, an allogeneic HLA-identical stem cell transplant was performed. During the

KARGER

E-Mail karger@karger.com
www.karger.com/drm

© 2016 S. Karger AG, Basel
1018–8665/16/2327–0009$39.50/0

Dr. med. Carlo Mainetti
Department of Dermatology
Ospedale Regionale Bellinzona e Valli
CH–6500 Bellinzona (Switzerland)
E-Mail info@carlomainetti.ch

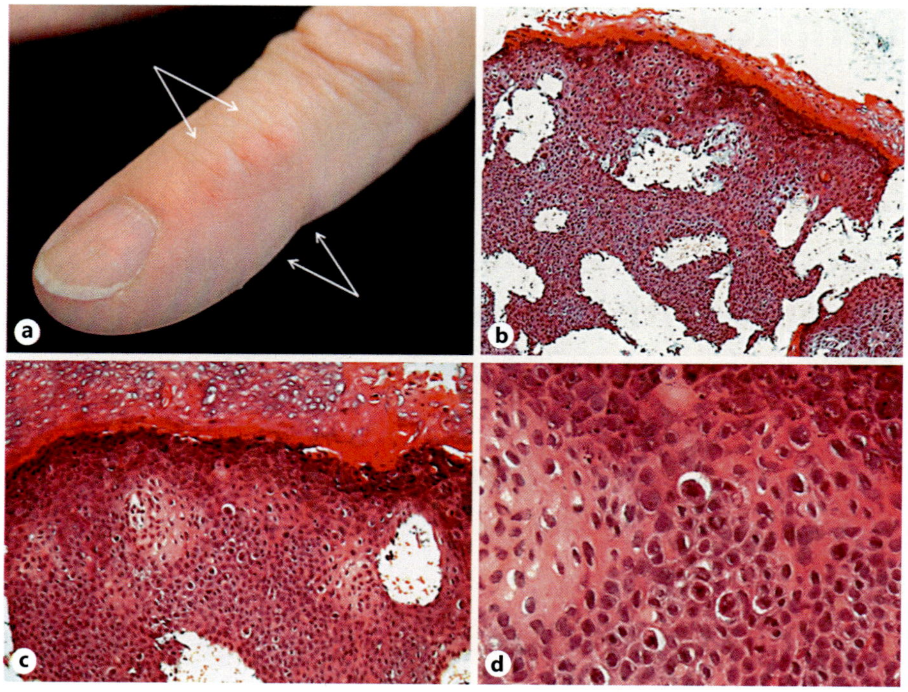

Fig. 1. a Relapsing BD of the right forefinger 5 years after the first diagnosis; **b** shave-excision with full-thickness atypia of the epidermis and parakeratosis. H&E ×100; **c** disorderly maturation of the epidermis with marked atypia and dyskeratotic cells. H&E ×200; **d** dyskeratotic cells and mitoses at different levels in the epidermis. H&E ×400.

2 years after the bone marrow transplant, the patient benefitted from immunosuppressive therapy with oral cyclosporine A. In the following years, she no longer needed any treatment for her hematological disease and did not experience relapse throughout this period. The patient's state of health was satisfactory except that 7 years after the bone marrow transplant she developed an adenocarcinoma of the right lung lower lobe (stage γpT3 γpNO MO), which was successfully removed by right lower pulmonary lobectomy.

One year after stem cell transplant and 9 years after the initial diagnosis, she slowly developed an erythematous plaque on her right forefinger. A skin biopsy was performed and the histological diagnosis was BD. A 5-fluorouracil (5-FU) 5% cream applied twice daily for 3 weeks led to remission of BD, but less than a year later, she relapsed. During the following years, BD was treated with different modalities alternating between 5-FU and imiquimod (IQ) 5% gel, always relapsing a few months after every treatment cycle. This cycle of remission and relapse continued after cyclosporine A had been stopped as well.

We examined the patient for the first time 15 years after the first diagnosis of myeloproliferative syndrome and 6 years after the stem cell transplant. On the distal medial aspect of her right forefinger, she presented an erythematous plaque that overflowed above the line of Wallace measuring 15 × 12 mm (fig. 1a). We performed a shave biopsy in truncal anesthesia. The histological examination confirmed the diagnosis of BD showing full thickness, markedly atypical and dyskeratotic cells of epidermis with mitoses and parakeratosis (fig. 1b–d). Afterward, the patient was treated by a methyl aminolaevulinate (MAL) – photodynamic therapy (PDT). BD relapsed at the lesion edges after 6 months. We therefore treated with IQ 5% cream for 1 month, but BD recurred again 6 months thereafter. One year after the first MAL-PDT, it was treated for a second time.

After a year's relapse of BD at the edges (fig. 2a, b), we decided to perform an off-label treatment with IM 500 μg/g gel, administered once daily for 2 consecutive days, following the clinical course with dermoscopy. At that moment, a treatment with 5-FU 5% cream was refused by the patient, because she complained of pain during previous therapies. Three days after the first application of IM, the skin lesions occurred more reddening and vesicular (fig. 2c). At the dermoscopy examination, the typical glomerular vessels had disappeared, leaving room for an apple juice-like colored picture without vascular structures (fig. 2d). But after 6 weeks, the clinical appearance seemed to have reverted to the same state as before the treatment, which was also confirmed by a dermoscopy where glomerular vessels in the lesion reappeared (fig. 3a, b). With the informed consent of the patient, we decided to treat her with IM 500 μg/g gel, administered once daily for 1 day under occlusion of a patch. The patient complained of pain and a burning sensation a few hours after application of IM. We treated with oral paracetamol 3 times 1 g daily. Following the removal of the patch after 24 h, the symptoms disappeared gradually after 2 days. Three days after the application of IM, vesicular and dyshidrotic skin lesions occurred (fig. 3c). On dermoscopy, the lesions showed a scaly and hyperkeratotic picture with disappearance of the glomerular vessels (fig. 3d). At 6 weeks follow-up, we found clinical remission (fig. 4a) without glomerular vessels on dermoscopy (fig. 4b). Follow-up at 3 months confirmed clinical and dermoscopical remission (fig. 4c, d). At 6 months' follow-up after the second treatment with IM, there had been no relapse with excellent cosmesis.

Discussion

Cutaneous BD is an intra-epidermal skin tumor, presenting as a circumscribed erythematous plaque with scaly or crusted surface or as verrucous or pigmented

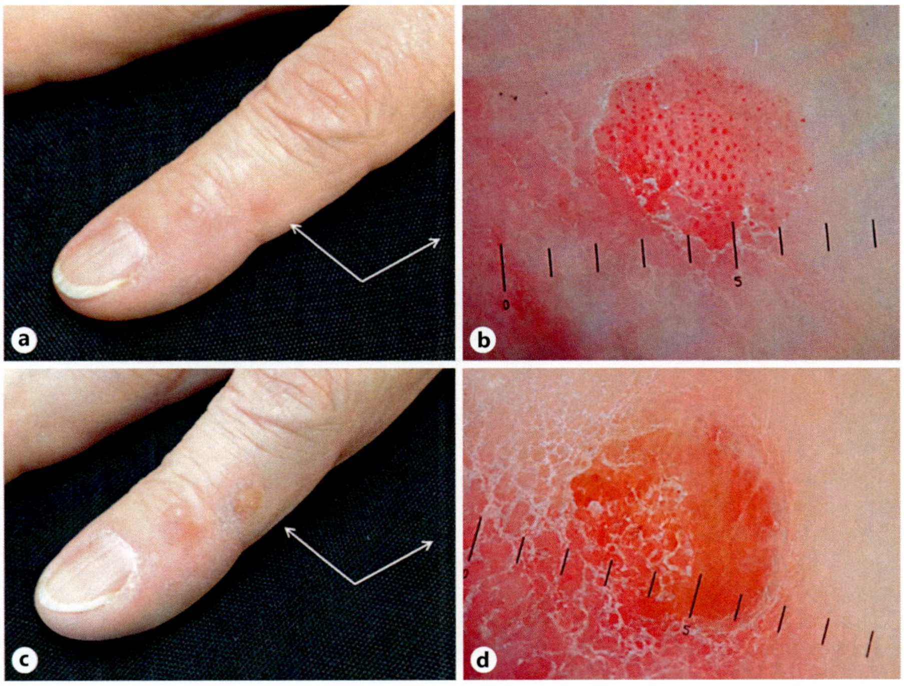

Fig. 2. a Relapsing BD of the right forefinger 8 years after the first diagnosis; **b** dermoscopy of non-pigmented BD showing glomerular vessels that are arranged in clusters and white to yellow scales; **c** after 3 days' treatment with IM, moderate-to-severe reaction is visible with confluent dyshidrotic vesicles; **d** dermoscopy after 3 days' treatment with IM, amorphous erythematous confluent vesicles and white scales.

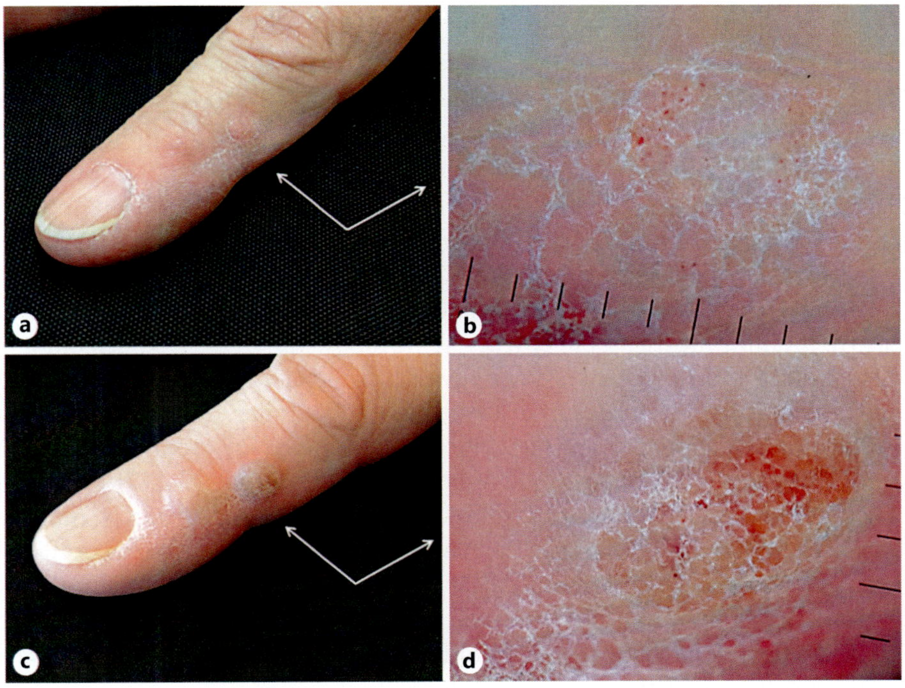

Fig. 3. a Relapsing BD of the right forefinger 6 weeks after the first IM treatment; **b** dermoscopy showing a resurgence of dotted and glomerular vessels associated with marketed white scales; **c** after 3 days' treatment with IM, severe reaction is visible with confluent dyshidrotic vesicles; **d** dermoscopy after 3 days' treatment with IM, amorphous erythematous confluent vesicles and white scales.

variants. The risk of progression to an invasive SCC is small, estimated at 3–5%. Women are most affected (75–85% of the cases). About 3 quarters of tumors are localized in lower extremities. In 80–90% of the patients, the lesion appears solitary. Many etiological factors are discussed: irradiation (solar, photochemotherapy, radiotherapy), arsenic, immunosuppressive diseases or treatments, chronic dermatoses or pre-existent skin lesions and viral-oncogenic human papilloma virus. About 30–50% of the subjects, who developed a BD, also develop or

Dermatology 2016;232(suppl 1):9–13
DOI: 10.1159/000447389

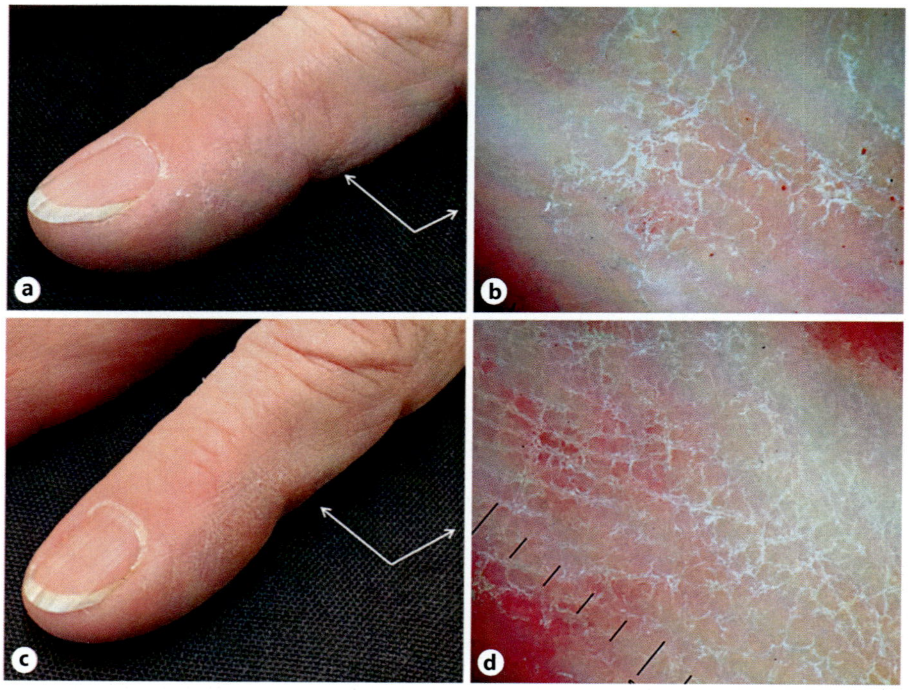

Fig. 4. a The right forefinger 6 weeks after the second IM treatment; **b** dermoscopy not showing a resurgence of dotted and glomerular vessels. White scales; **c** after 3 months' treatment with IM, no BD relapse is visible; **d** dermoscopy after 3 months' treatment with IM, not showing a resurgence of dotted and glomerular vessels.

have developed a non-melanoma skin cancer, probably reflecting common solar damage [1, 2, 8].

The clinical diagnosis of BD is usually confirmed by a biopsy, showing full-thickness epidermal dysplasia without dermal invasion [1, 2, 8]. Micali et al. [9] reviewed, according to evidence-based analysis, therapeutic possibilities for the topical treatment of skin cancers and found 5-FU, IQ, PDT and surgery with documented efficacy.

Dermoscopy is used by dermatologists not only as a non-invasive method for the diagnosis of skin cancers but also to monitor the treatment efficacy in the follow-up. At dermoscopy, non-pigmented BD shows a characteristic morphologic type of dotted and tortuous vessels similar to the glomerular apparatus of the kidneys or arranged in lines at the periphery and opaque, yellow to white scales. Histopathologically, the glomerular vessels correspond to the presence of convolutions of capillaries in the dermal papillae, which are grouped in clusters and are dilated [3, 4, 10–13]. Mun et al. [4] proposed an algorithm for the clinical use of dermoscopy to monitor the therapeutic response of BD: once these vascular structures disappear, the BD is clinically cured. The histopathological examination typically is negative for remains of BD. In these cases, the authors suggested a regular follow-up by dermoscopy. If on dermoscopy the glomerular vessels persist, a histopathological assessment of the skin lesion is needed, and in these cases, BD is typically found on histology [4].

In Australia, Ogbourne et al. [14] first described the preclinical activity of IM (PEP005, ingenol-3-angelate), a hydrophobic diterpene ester isolated from the plant *Euphorbia peplus*, for the treatment of skin cancer. The same group demonstrated that IM field-directed treatment of UVB-damaged skin reduced tumor lesion formation and removed mutant p53 patches [15]. A recent article elucidated direct effects of IM on primary keratinocytes, patient-derived SCC cells and a SCC cell line [16]. IM thus inhibits viability and proliferation of all keratinocyte-derived cells in a biphasic way – IM-induced cell death is mediated through the PKCδ/MEK/ERK pathway and the downstream induction of IL1R2 and IL13RA2 expression to the reduced viability of IM-treated cells [16]. Longo et al. [17] recently reported 2 cases of non-invasive monitoring of morphological changes in AK treated with IM using a combination of dermoscopy and reflectance confocal microscopy. They concluded that both methods represent a non-invasive possibility to monitor treatment efficacy of this new drug [17].

We describe a case of recurring BD successfully treated with IM gel. A first article [18] reported a case of a 74-year-old man treated with sunitinib, a multi-kinase inhibitor, for metastatic renal cell carcinoma that he had developed together with numerous SCC and 2 BD tumors at his abdomen. He was treated with IM gel 0.05% once daily for 2 days consecutively. The healing was confirmed by histopathological examination, but was only partial in 1 of the 2 BD tumors. The authors wrote that a second treatment cycle was planned. A second article [19] reported a case of a 79-year-old woman with BD on the right calf. The authors applied IM 0.05% gel on the tumor area once daily for 3 days consecutively, achieving a total remission after 10 weeks, confirmed by histopathological examination and without recurrence 6 months after treatment.

Our patient's BD had developed when she was still under pharmacological immunosuppression with cyclosporine A. Her immunosuppression may well have been an aggravating factor in the numerous recurrences observed. As in the first reported case [18], remission occurred after occlusive use of IM. We thus propose that for recalcitrant or relapsing cases of BD, occlusive treatment with IM may be a promising approach. Serial dermoscopy proved a helpful procedure informing about treatment outcome with early detection of relapse at 6 weeks after the first application of IM and sparing the patient from additional biopsies. We thus believe that dermoscopy is a valuable method for the follow-up of topical treatments in BD treated with IM [3, 4, 11–13, 17].

Funding

This study did not receive funding from third parties.

Statement of Ethics

Informed consent was obtained from the patient.

Disclosure Statement

C.G. and S.L.-P. declare that they have no conflicts of interest. C.M. is member of the Advisory Board Dermatology for LEO Pharma.

References

1 Cox NH, Eedy DJ, Morton CA; Therapy Guidelines and Audit Subcommittee, British Association of Dermatologists: Guidelines for management of Bowen's disease: 2006 update. Br J Dermatol 2007;156:11–21.

2 Morton CA, Birnie AJ, Eedy DJ: British association of dermatologists' guidelines for the management of squamous cell carcinoma in situ (Bowen's disease) 2014. Br J Dermatol 2014;170:245–260.

3 Zalaudek I, Argenziano G, Leinweber B, Citarella L, Hofmann-Wellenhof R, Malvehy J, Puig S, Pizzichetta MA, Thomas L, Soyer HP, Kerl H: Dermoscopy of Bowen's disease. Br J Dermatol 2004;150:1112–1116.

4 Mun JH, Park JM, Song M, Jwa SW, Kim HS, Ko HC, Kim BS, Kim MB: The use of dermatoscopy to monitor therapeutic response of Bowen disease: a dermatoscopic pathological study. Br J Dermatol 2012;167:1382–1385.

5 Hofbauer G, Anliker M, Boehncke WH, Brand C, Braun R, Gaide O, Hafner J, Hunger R, Itin P, Kaeuper G, Lautenschlager S, Mainetti C, Streit M: Swiss clinical practice guidelines on field cancerization of the skin. Swiss Med Wkly 2014;144:w14026.

6 Rosen RH, Gupta AK, Tyring SK: Dual mechanism of action of ingenol mebutate gel for topical treatment of actinic keratoses: rapid lesion necrosis followed by lesion-specific immune response. J Am Acad Dermatol 2012; 66:486–493.

7 Lebwohl M, Swanson N, Anderson LL, Melgaard A, Xu Z, Berman B: Ingenol mebutate gel for actinic keratosis. N Engl J Med 2012; 366:1010–1019.

8 Morley GL, Matthews JH, Verpetinske I, Thom GA: A comparative study examining the management of Bowen's disease in the United Kingdom and Australia. Dermatol Res Pract 2015;2015:421460.

9 Micali G, Lacarrubba F, Nasca MR, Ferraro S, Schwartz RA: Topical pharmacotherapy for skin cancer: part II. Clinical applications. J Am Acad Dermatol 2014;70:979.e1–e12.

10 Argenziano G, Zalaudek I, Corona R, Sera F, Cicale L, Petrillo G, Ruocco E, Hofmann-Wellenhof R, Soyer HP: Vascular structures in skin tumors: a dermoscopy study. Arch Dermatol 2004;140:1485–1489.

11 Zalaudek I, Di Stefani A, Argenziano G: The specific dermoscopic criteria of Bowen's disease. J Eur Acad Dermatol Venereol 2006;20: 361–362.

12 Payapvipapong K, Tanaka M: Corona of glomerular vessels: a diagnostic marker of hyperkeratotic Bowen's disease. Dermatol Surg 2013;39:1395–1398.

13 Zalaudek I, Argenziano G: Dermoscopy of actinic keratosis, intraepidermal carcinoma and squamous cell carcinoma. Curr Probl Dermatol 2015;46:70–76.

14 Ogbourne SM, Suhrbier A, Jones B, Cozzi SJ, Boyle GM, Morris M, McAlpine D, Johns J, Scott TM, Sutherland KP, Gardner JM, Le TT, Lenarczyk A, Aylward JH, Parsons PG: Antitumor activity of 3-ingenyl angelate: plasma membrane and mitochondrial disruption and necrotic cell death. Cancer Res 2004;64:2833–2839.

15 Cozzi SJ, Ogbourne SM, James C, Rebel HG, de Gruijl FR, Ferguson B, Gardner J, Lee TT, Larcher T, Suhrbier A: Ingenol mebutate field-directed treatment of UVB-damaged skin reduces lesion formation and removes mutant p53 patches. J Invest Dermatol 2012; 132:1263–1271.

16 Freiberger SN, Cheng PF, Iotzova-Weiss G, Neu J, Liu Q, Dziunycz P, Zibert JR, Dummer R, Skak K, Levesque MP, Hofbauer GF: Ingenol mebutate signals via PKC/MEK/ERK in keratinocytes and induces interleukin decoy receptors IL1R2 and IL13RA2. Mol Cancer Ther 2015;14:2132–2142.

17 Longo C, Borsari S, Benati E, Moscarella E, Alfano R, Argenziano G: Dermoscopy and reflectance confocal microscopy for monitoring the treatment of actinic keratosis with ingenol mebutate gel: report of two cases. Dermatol Ther (Heidelb) 2016;6:81–87.

18 Braun SA, Homey B, Gerber PA: [Successful treatment of Bowen disease with ingenol mebutate]. Hautarzt 2014;65:848–850.

19 Lee JH, Lee JH, Bae JM, Kim GM: Successful treatment of Bowen's disease with ingenol mebutate 0.05% gel. J Dermatol 2015;42:920–921.

Dermatology

Dermatology 2016;232(suppl 1):14–16
DOI: 10.1159/000447390

Published online: August 11, 2016

Bowenoid Actinic Keratosis and Bowen's Disease Treated Successfully with Ingenol Mebutate

Mosab T. Mohanna[a, b] Günther F.L. Hofbauer[a]

[a]Department of Dermatology, University Hospital Zurich, Zurich, Switzerland; [b]Department of Dermatology, Taibah University, Medina, Saudi Arabia

Key Words

Actinic keratosis · Bowen's disease · Ingenol mebutate

Abstract

Ingenol mebutate (IM) is a topical pharmacotherapy approved in Switzerland since 2012 for treating non-hypertrophic, non-hyperkeratotic actinic keratosis (AK). We report 2 cases with off-label use of IM. The first case of bowenoid AK was treated with 150 μg IM for 3 consecutive days with an almost complete clinical remission of the lesion. The second case of Bowen's disease was treated with 500 μg IM for 2 consecutive days leading to complete clinical remission.

© 2016 S. Karger AG, Basel

Case Report

We report on the use of ingenol mebutate (IM) in bowenoid actinic keratosis (AK) and Bowen's disease (BD), both of which are beyond the registered indication of non-hypertrophic, non-hyperplastic AK and thus constitute off-label treatment.

Case One

The first case was a 78-year-old female patient referred to our clinic for a histologically confirmed bowenoid AK at the lateral commissure of her lower left eyelid. Various topical modalities including imiquimod (IQ) and photodynamic therapy (PDT) had been performed with varying success. Due to the size and location of the lesion, the service of plastic surgery declined total excision, which corresponded to patient preference as well. Based on a phase I/II clinical study using *Euphorbia peplus* sap with the active ingredient IM in treating intra-epidermal carcinomas (IECs) successfully in a limited number of patients [1], we decided to apply 150 μg IM for 3 consecutive days as off-label treatment for this bowenoid AK. A pronounced local skin reaction around the left eye with erythema and erosion was seen, with disappearance of pigmentation and remaining erythema without scaling at 2 weeks of follow-up. Dermatoscopically, focal peppering with almost complete clinical regression of the pigmentation was seen at 6-month follow-up with good cosmetic outcome (fig. 1).

Case Two

The second case was a 73-year-old male patient in regular follow-up in our clinic for a history of dermatitis who presented with a new skin lesion on the left dorsum of the hand. Clinically, a brown-red plaque of 2 cm diameter was observed. Dermatoscopically, a pseudo-network, superficial scales and dotted vessels were noted. Based on our clinical diagnosis of BD and on our successful treatment of the first case with bowenoid AK as well as the patient's desire of a simplified way of treatment, we started an off-label treatment with 500 μg IM for 2 consecutive days, leading to crust formation, which resolved after 1 week with complete clinical remission at 6 weeks' follow-up (fig. 2).

Discussion

BD is a form of squamous cell carcinoma in-situ, which may develop to invasive SCC in 3–26% cases when left untreated [2]. Surgical excision, laser destruction, electroco-

KARGER

E-Mail karger@karger.com
www.karger.com/drm

© 2016 S. Karger AG, Basel
1018–8665/16/2327–0014$39.50/0

Mosab T. Mohanna, MD
Department of Dermatology, University Hospital Zurich
Gloriastrasse 31
CH–8091 Zurich (Switzerland)
E-Mail mohanna.mosabtariq@usz.ch

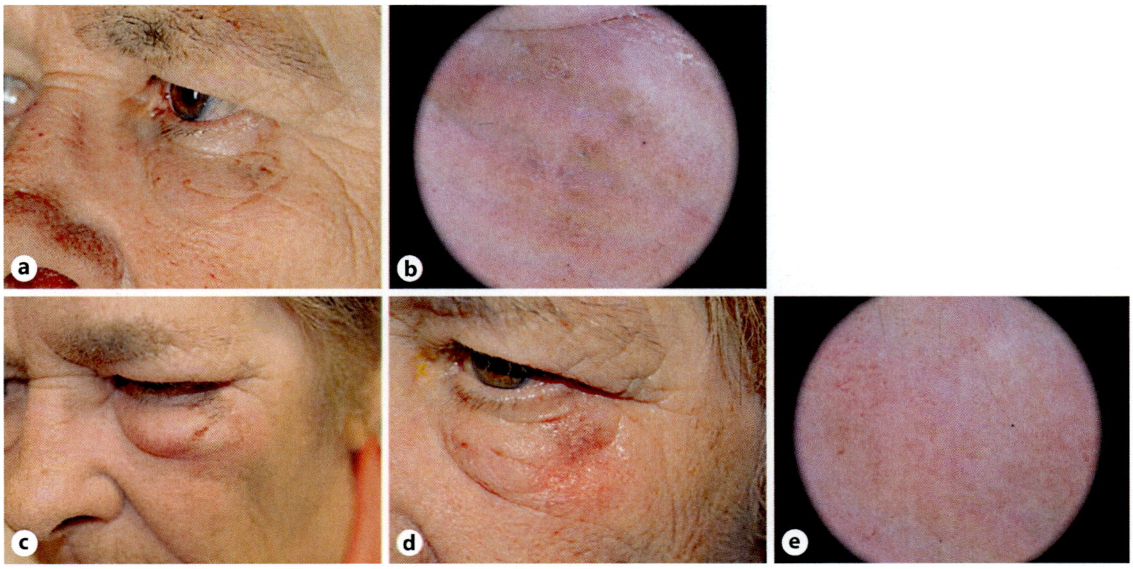

Fig. 1. a A brown macule at the lateral corner of the left eye was histologically confirmed as bowenoid AK. **b** Dermatoscopic picture of the lesion shows hyperkeratosis, brown pigmentation and focal peppering with telangiectasia. **c** A pronounced local skin reaction around the left eye with erythema and erosion formed after applying 150 μg IM for 3 consecutive days. **d** A marked improvement of pigmented AK, without infiltration, but a remaining erythema at 2 weeks after IM. **e** Dermatoscopic picture after IM shows a disappearing of the hyperkeratosis, pigmentation and peppering with telangiectasia.

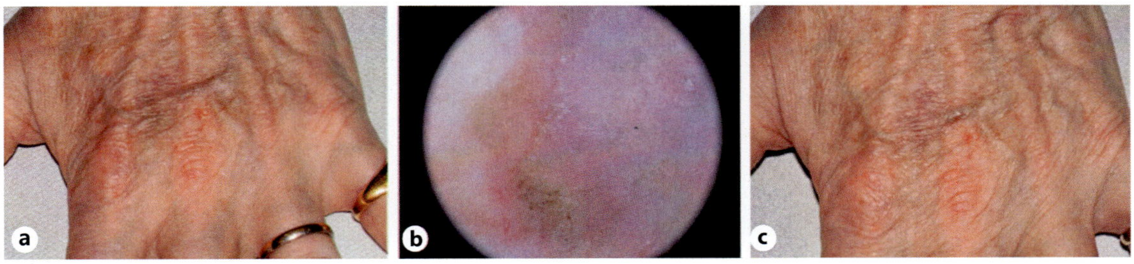

Fig. 2. a Two centimeters hyperkeratotic brown-red plaque on the dorsum of left hand. **b** Dermatoscopic picture of the lesion shows a pseudo-network, superficial scales and dotted vessels. **c** A post-inflammatory macule after treatment using 500 μg IM for 2 consequence days with clinical remission at 6 weeks.

agulation and desiccation and cryosurgery are accepted ablative treatment options [2]. Therapeutic alternatives to surgery include PDT [3], radiotherapy and topical treatments such as 5-fluorouracil and IQ [4]. Most topical pharmacotherapies induce inflammation with long application period ranging from weeks to months. IM is an active compound in the sap of *Euphorbia peplus* and has 2 mechanisms of action, including necrosis within hours and cellular cytotoxicity within days, making it a very rapid topical treatment modality [1, 5]. IM has been registered in the United States, the European Union and in Switzerland as a treatment for AK since 2012 [5]. One advantage of using IM is the short treating course, which could improve patient compliance [1, 4, 5]. A clinical study with *Euphorbia peplus* sap with an active ingredient IM (PEP005) showed that the effectiveness of IM is not limited to superficial AK only but also extends to clinical healing of IEC in 94% of patients studied [1]. A case reported was published in September 2014 on successful treatment of multiple BD by IM in a patient on systemic treatment with the multikinase inhibitor sunitinib for metastatic clear-cell renal carcinoma [6]. In our case, the same treatment regimen of AK using IM was applied and led to a successful clinical improvement and remission with high patient satisfaction.

In conclusion, IM could be a useful topical treatment option off-label for patients with BD or hypertrophic, hyperkeratotic AK with the hallmarks of short duration and easy self-application.

Statement of Ethics

We do not have the patients' consent since they were treated more than 2–3 years ago, and in one case there was no follow-up.

Disclosure Statement

The publication costs of this report were financially supported by LEO Pharma.

References

1 Ramsay JR, Suhrbier A, Aylward JH, Ogbourne S, Cozzi SJ, Poulsen MG, Baumann KC, Welburn P, Redlich GL, Parsons PG: The sap from Euphorbia peplus is effective against human nonmelanoma skin cancers. Br J Dermatol 2011;164:633–636.

2 Micali G, Lacarrubba F, Nasca MR, Ferraro S, Schwartz RA: Topical pharmacotherapy for skin cancer: part II. Clinical applications. J Am Acad Dermatol 2014;70:979.e1–e12; quiz 9912.

3 Westers-Attema A, Lohman BG, van den Heijkant F, Nelemans PJ, Winnepenninckx VJ, Kelleners-Smeets NW, Mosterd K: Photodynamic therapy in Bowen's disease: influence of histological features and clinical characteristics on its success. Dermatology 2015;230:55–61.

4 Lucena SR, Salazar N, Gracia-Cazaña T, Zamarrón A, González S, Juarranz Á, Gilaberte Y: Combined treatments with photodynamic therapy for non-melanoma skin cancer. Int J Mol Sci 2015;16:25912–25933.

5 Mohanna M, Hofbauer G: Pronounced local skin reaction to ingenol mebutate against actinic keratosis in kidney transplant recipient without systemic adverse events. JAAD Case Rep 2015;1:S19–S22.

6 Braun SA, Homey B, Gerber PA: [Successful treatment of Bowen disease with ingenol mebutate]. Hautarzt 2014;65:848–850.

Dermatology

Dermatology 2016;232(suppl 1):17–19
DOI: 10.1159/000447391

Published online: August 11, 2016

Ingenol Mebutate 150 mg as Physician-Directed Treatment of Bowen's Disease Under Occlusion

Ahmed Alkhalaf[a, b] Günther F.L. Hofbauer[a]

[a]Department of Dermatology, University Hospital Zurich, Zurich, Switzerland; [b]Department of Dermatology, University Hospital Al-Majmaah, Al-Majmaah, Saudi Arabia

Key Words
Ingenol mebutate · Bowen's disease · Photodynamic therapy

Abstract
Ingenol mebutate (IM) is a topical pharmacotherapy approved in Switzerland since 2012 for treating non-hypertrophic, non-hyperkeratotic actinic keratosis. We report a case with off-label use of IM where Bowen's disease has been successfully treated with physician-directed IM 0.015% gel under occlusion over the chest area. © 2016 S. Karger AG, Basel

Introduction

Bowen's disease is an in-situ squamous cell carcinoma of the skin with approximately 3–5% of risk of progression to invasive carcinoma [1]. Although surgical excision is the definitive treatment, non-surgical treatment modalities including photodynamic therapy, 5-fluorouracil and imiquimod are effective alternatives for Bowen's disease, especially in patients who are poor candidates for surgery [2]. Judging by clinical experience, Bowen's disease is harder to treat than actinic keratosis. We herein report a case of Bowen's disease successfully treated with physician-directed ingenol mebutate (IM) 0.015% gel under occlusion over the chest area.

Case Report

We describe the case of a 82-year-old Caucasian man, Fitzpatrick skin type II, followed up at our clinic for a history of severe sun-damaged skin, actinic keratosis and multiple keratinocyte skin cancers.

The patient presented with 4 shiny red, well-demarcated plaques with/without scaling on the chest. Dermoscopy showed a clear pattern of dotted vessels. Based on the clinical and the dermatoscopical appearance of the lesions, a diagnosis of multiple Bowen's disease was made (fig. 1).

Based on the patient's preference for non-surgical treatment, we presented him with different topical treatment options. As the mobility of his hands was limited following orthopedic surgery, a physician-directed treatment was needed. Photodynamic therapy was declined by the patient on account of the expected pain associated with the procedure. Cryotherapy was deemed less suitable due to the number of lesions and potentially long wound healing. We decided to use IM as a physician-directed treatment, employing an occlusive dressing to enable a single application to elicit a thera-

KARGER

E-Mail karger@karger.com
www.karger.com/drm

© 2016 S. Karger AG, Basel
1018–8665/16/2327–0017$39.50/0

Dr. Ahmed Alkhalaf
Department of Dermatology, University Hospital Zurich
Gloriastrasse 31
CH–8091 Zurich (Switzerland)
E-Mail Ahmed.Alkhalaf@usz.ch

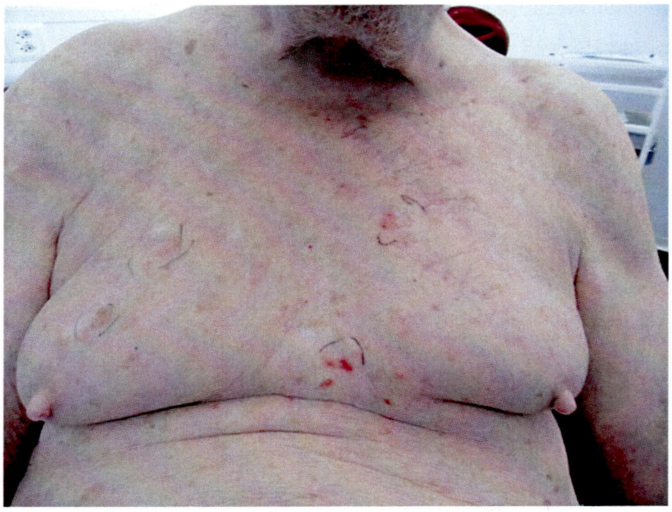

Fig. 1. 4 shiny red, well-demarcated plaques with/without scaling on the chest. Dermoscopy showed a clear pattern of dotted vessels treated with 150 μg IM gel on each lesion with a surface area of around 2 × 2 cm to extend 5 mm beyond the lesion. The treatment area was then covered with a waterproof bandage for 1 day to assess the local skin response under occlusion.

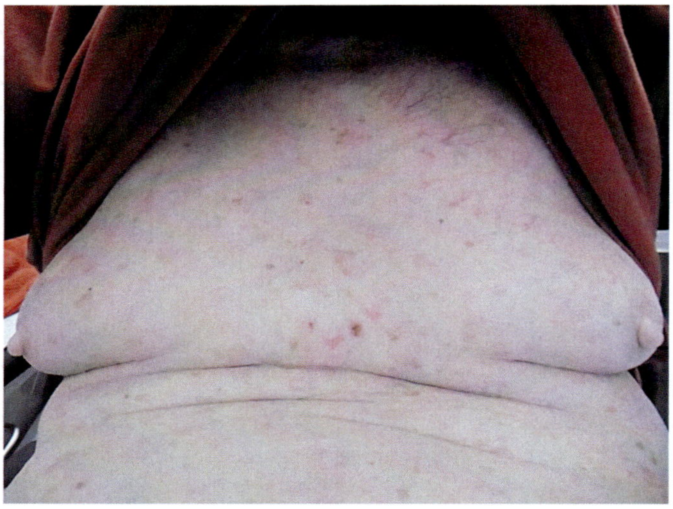

Fig. 2. At 6-month follow-up, 2 lesions of Bowen's disease went into clinical remission. Two lesions of BD persisted and were again treated as described above for 2 days under occlusion.

peutic local response. As we expected an increased local skin reaction due to occlusive application, we chose the lower of the 2 concentrations of IM available for this off-label treatment. We directly applied 150 μg IM gel on each lesion with a surface area of around 2 × 2 cm to extend 5 mm beyond the lesion. The treatment area was then covered with a waterproof bandage for 1 day to assess the local skin response under occlusion. At the same time, we used cryotherapy on one circumscribed, clinically diagnosed non-hypertrophic actinic keratosis over the right temporal area. Starting on the third day, the patient experienced erythema extending beyond the application site, pain within the area of application, which he reported as similar to what he perceived in the right temporal area treated with cryotherapy. The local skin reaction on the chest lasted almost 2 weeks. No systemic symptoms such as fever, chills, fatigue or malaise were reported. At 3-month follow-up, we repeated the treatment at our office on the 4 lesions of BD. This time, we asked the patient to keep the bandage on for 2 days because the lesions had persisted. At 6-month follow-up, 2 lesions of Bowen's disease went into clinical remission (fig. 2). Two lesions of BD persisted and were again treated as described above for 2 days under occlusion (fig. 2).

Discussion

In Switzerland, registered non-surgical treatments for BD include topical 5-fluorouracil, photodynamic therapy and cryotherapy. Topical 5-fluorouracil 5% cream clinically cured 85% of patients in one small, uncontrolled study, administered twice daily for an average of 8 weeks (average follow-up time = 4.6 years) [3]. The efficacy of PDT for Bowen's disease was illustrated by a randomized trial in which 225 patients were randomly assigned to PDT with MAL (MAL-PDT), PDT using a placebo or conventional treatment (either cryotherapy or topical 5-FU). The lesion recurrence rates at 12 months were similar with MAL-PDT, cryotherapy and topical 5-FU (15, 21 and 17%, respectively) [4]. Cryotherapy appears to have a good success rate for Bowen's disease with adequate treatment (recurrences less than 10% at 12 months) but healing may be slow for broad lesions and discomfort may limit treatment of multiple lesions. Curettage and PDT both have higher success rates and less discomfort overall, but are more time-consuming and/or expensive to perform [5]. A systematic review of observational studies that identified 8 studies (with a total of 273 patients) that assessed recurrence rates for invasive cutaneous SCC after cryotherapy found a pooled average recurrence rate of 0.8% (95% CI 0.1–2.2) [6].

Frequently used as off-label treatment for BD in Switzerland, imiquimod cured BD at a rate between 73 and 88% in one small, randomized trial and several small, uncontrolled studies [7].

IM is a topical drug extract from the latex sap of a plant *Euphorbia peplus* that acts by chemo-ablative and immune-stimulatory properties [8]. Its dual mechanism of action consists of a rapid induction of inflammation with primary necrosis of tumor cells, followed by neutrophil-mediated, antibody-dependent cellular cytotoxicity of residual cells [9]. The Food and Drug Administration ap-

Dermatology 2016;232(suppl 1):17–19
DOI: 10.1159/000447391

proved IM for therapy of actinic keratosis in 2012 [10]. One case report from South Korea and one from Germany describe successful treatment of Bowen's disease outside the facial area with IM 0.05%. The South Korean report had used IM 0.05% once daily for 3 days consecutively on one lesion over the right calf. Ten weeks after treatment, clinical remission was confirmed histologically by multiple punch biopsies without evidence of BD [11]. The German case used IM 0.05% once daily for 2 days consecutively on 2 lesions. At 2-month follow-up, one lesion was clinically resolved confirmed by punch biopsy, while the second lesion needed retreatment [12]. Intra-epidermal carcinomas were clinically healed in 94% of patients in a clinical study employing *Euphorbia peplus* sap with IM (previously labeled as PEP005) [13].

Our case report adds to the data on treatment of BD using IM. Our treatment protocol with a single application at the time of consultation in our clinic allowed using IM as a one-time intervention akin to PDT. In contrast to PDT, our treatment with IM was rapid and without immediate pain. The use of an occlusive dressing, although officially not recommended, may be a benefit when turning IM from a self-directed into a physician-directed treatment, addressing the needs of an elderly population and of anatomical sites difficult to access in self-directed treatment.

Statement of Ethics

Patient consent was obtained.

Disclosure Statement

The publication costs for this case report were supported by LEO Pharma.

References

1 Jaeger AB, Gramkow A, Hjalgrim H, Melbye M, Frisch M: Bowen disease and risk of subsequent malignant neoplasms: a population-based cohort study of 1147 patients. Arch Dermatol 1999;135:790–793.
2 Bonerandi JJ, Beauvillain C, Caquant L, et al: French Dermatology Recommendations Association (aRED): Guidelines for the diagnosis and treatment of cutaneous squamous cell carcinoma and precursor lesions. J Eur Acad Dermatol Venereol 2011;25(suppl 5): 1–51.
3 Bargman H, Hochman J: Topical treatment of Bowen's disease with 5-fluorouracil. J Cutan Med Surg 2003;7:101.
4 Morton C, Horn M, Leman J, et al: Comparison of topical methyl aminolevulinate photodynamic therapy with cryotherapy or fluorouracil for treatment of squamous cell carcinoma in situ: results of a multicenter randomized trial. Arch Dermatol 2006;142: 729–735.
5 Cox NH, Eedy DJ, Morton CA: Guidelines for management of Bowen's disease: 2006 update. Br J Dermatol 2007;156:11–21.
6 Lansbury L, Bath-Hextall F, Perkins W, et al: Interventions for non-metastatic squamous cell carcinoma of the skin: systematic review and pooled analysis of observational studies. BMJ 2013;347:f6153.
7 Love WE, Bernhard JD, Bordeaux JS: Topical imiquimod or fluorouracil therapy for basal and squamous cell carcinoma: a systematic review. Arch Dermatol 2009;145:1431–1438.
8 Fallen RS, Gooderham M: Ingenol mebutate: an introduction. Skin Therapy Lett 2012;17: 1–3.
9 Freiberger SN, et al: Ingenol mebutate signals via PKC/MEK/ERK in keratinocytes and induces interleukin decoy receptors IL1R2 and IL13RA2. Mol Cancer Ther 2015;14:2132–2142.
10 Siller G, Rosen R, Freeman M, et al: PEP005 (ingenol mebutate) gel for the topical treatment of superficial basal cell carcinoma: results of a randomized phase IIa trial. Australas J Dermatol 2010;51:99–105.
11 Lee, JH, et al: Successful treatment of Bowen's disease with ingenol mebutate 0.05% gel. J Dermatol 2015;42:920–921.
12 Braun SA, Homey B, Gerber PA: Erfolgreiche Behandlung Eines Morbus Bowen Mit Ingenolmebutat. Hautarzt 2014;65:848–850.
13 Ramsay JR, Suhrbier A, Aylward JH, Ogbourne S, Cozzi SJ, Poulsen MG, Baumann KC, Welburn P, Redlich GL, Parsons PG: The sap from Euphorbia peplus is effective against human nonmelanoma skin cancers. Br J Dermatol 2011;164:633–636.

Dermatology

Dermatology 2016;232(suppl 1):20–23
DOI: 10.1159/000447392

Published online: August 11, 2016

Ingenol Mebutate vs. Daylight Photodynamic Therapy in a Kidney Transplant Recipient

Michael Mühlstädt

Division of Dermatology and Venerology, Geneva University Hospitals, Geneva, Switzerland

Key Words

Ingenol mebutate · Photodynamic therapy · Daylight photodynamic therapy · Methyl aminolevulinate · Field cancerization · Actinic keratosis · Immunosuppression

Abstract

We present the case of a 73-year-old male patient who had received a first renal transplant at 36 years and a second one at the age of 55 years. He is currently under immunosuppression with everolimus 2.5 mg/day and prednisone 5 mg/day. The patient presented with multiple actinic keratoses on both cheeks and the forehead and received treatment by ingenol mebutate 150 μg/g gel daily on 3 consecutive days on his right cheek and methyl aminolevulinate (MAL) photodynamic therapy activated by daylight (MAL-dPDT) on the forehead and the left cheek. MAL-dPDT treatment proved a feasible, repeatable, physician-directed method of treating field cancerization with limited morbidity for a period of 6 days. Treatment with ingenol mebutate gel was a feasible, possibly self-directed method of treating field cancerization with limited morbidity for 10 days in this immunosuppressed patient. Both treatments showed similar efficacy. At the time of treatment, the MAL daylight PDT ran at 3 times the cost of ingenol mebutate gel.

© 2016 S. Karger AG, Basel

This is the case of a 73-year-old male patient whom we follow on a regular basis in our outpatient clinic. At the age of 36 years, he received a first deceased-donor renal allograft for glomerular insufficiency of unknown origin and has been under continued immunosuppression ever since. Due to rejection of the first graft, he was transplanted a second time at the age of 55 years. Current immunosuppression employs everolimus 2.5 mg/day and prednisone 5 mg/day. The patient has a long-standing history of non-melanoma skin cancer including actinic keratoses, squamous cell carcinomas and basal cell carcinomas.

He has by now reached a state of pronounced field cancerization. Current guidelines prefer treatments that do not only remove a single lesion but will also address the already underlying cellular changes in its vicinity [1, 2]. Results of any one of these therapies may have a high inter-patient variability. For this reason, we chose 2 field-directed therapies – ingenol mebutate and photodynamic therapy (PDT) – in order to assess their individual efficacy in our patient.

We applied 150 μg/g ingenol mebutate gel once daily to the lesions on the right cheek on 3 consecutive days by respecting a maximum total surface area of 25 cm^2 as described in the official protocol of the drug [3]. Figure 1 shows the untreated right cheek, figure 2 shows the cheek

KARGER

E-Mail karger@karger.com
www.karger.com/drm

© 2016 S. Karger AG, Basel
1018–8665/16/2327–0020$39.50/0

Michael Mühlstädt
Division of Dermatology and Venerology, Geneva University Hospitals
Rue Gabrielle-Perret-Gentil 4
CH–1205 Geneva (Switzerland)
E-Mail mmuh@hcuge.ch

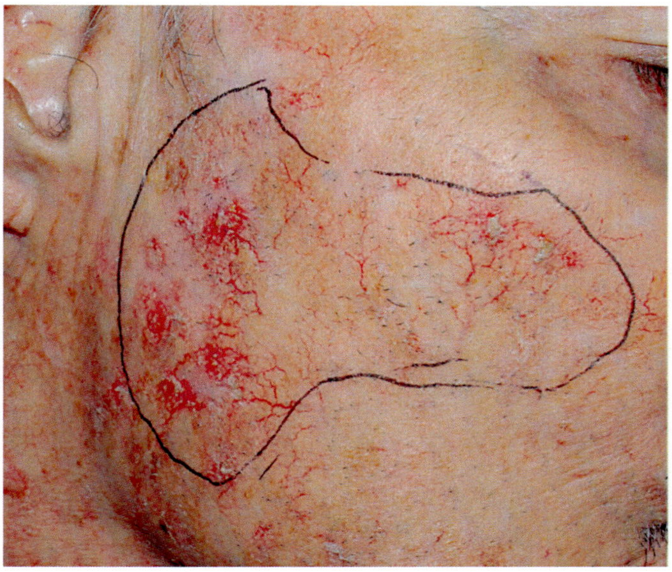

Fig. 1. Baseline of right cheek before treatment. The treatment area was marked with a pen. The patient left this labeling on for the 3 days of the treatment with ingenol mebutate.

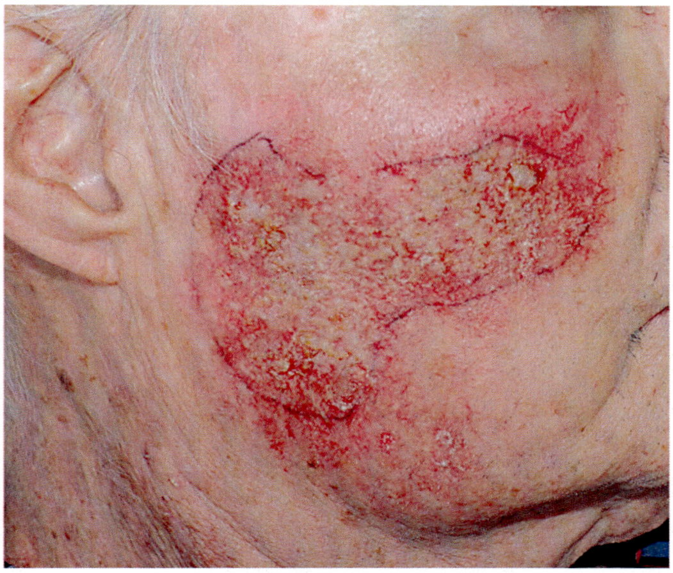

Fig. 2. Right cheek of the patient after 3 days of ingenol mebutate 150 μg/g once daily.

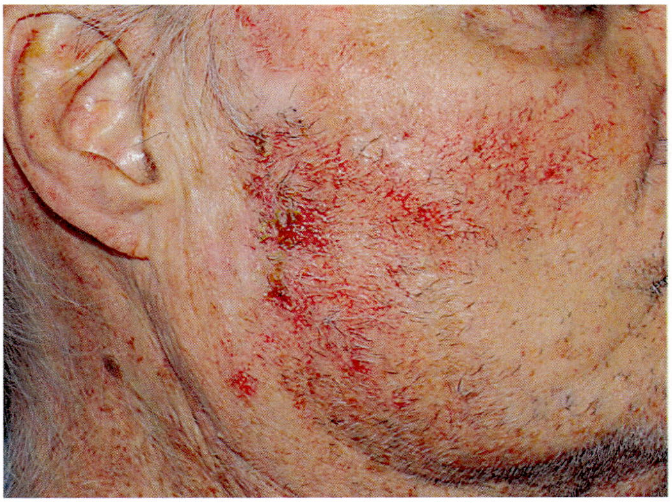

Fig. 3. Right cheek of the patient 10 days after the first application of ingenol mebutate 150 μg/g gel.

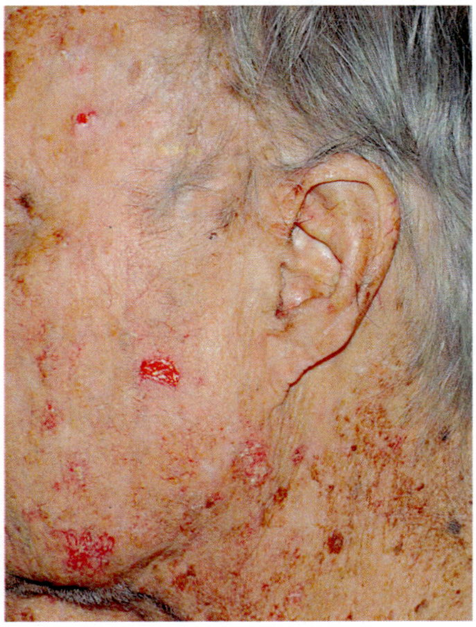

Fig. 4. Left cheek of the patient prior to MAL-dPDT treatment.

after 3 once daily applications of 150 μg/g ingenol mebutate gel as registered. A pustular reaction with crusts and erythema appeared in the gel treatment area. The patient reported only minor discomfort due to a mild burning sensation and had been informed about and consented orally to this not undesirable reaction beforehand. Ten days after the first application of ingenol mebutate 150 μg/g gel to the lesions on the right cheek, we saw the patient again (fig. 3). Erythema had almost returned to baseline.

On the same day, we conducted a treatment of daylight activated PDT with methyl aminolevulinate (MAL-dPDT) on the left cheek (fig. 4: baseline of the left cheek before MAL-dPDT treatment) according to the following

Dermatology 2016;232(suppl 1):20–23
DOI: 10.1159/000447392

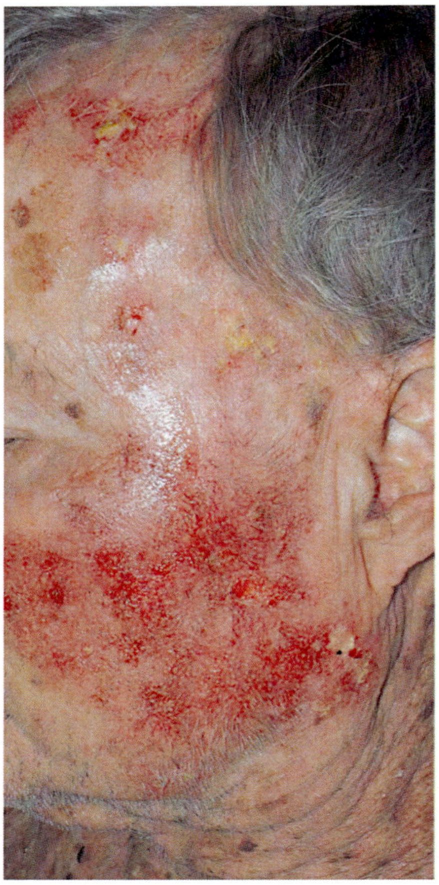

Fig. 5. Left cheek of the patient immediately after 2 h of MAL-dPDT treatment.

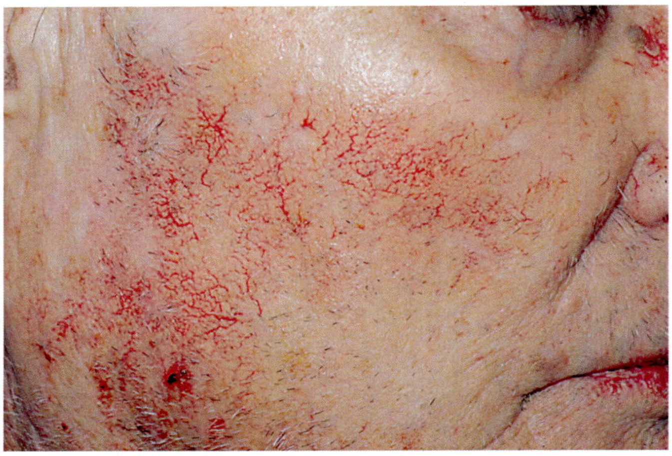

Fig. 6. Right cheek, 16 days after the beginning of a 3 days ingenol mebutate 150 µg/g gel treatment.

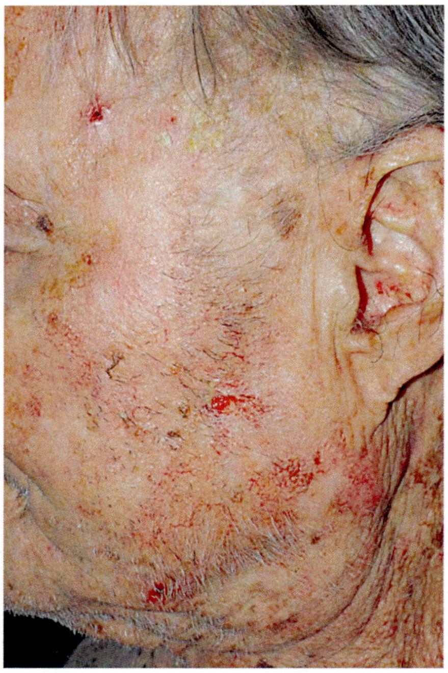

Fig. 7. Left cheek, 6 days after MAL-dPDT treatment.

protocol [4] – we applied chemical sunscreen to the face of the patient. After 30 min, the hyperkeratotic lesions (actinic keratoses) on the left cheek and the forehead were prepared by light curettage. Then MAL 16% was applied on the left cheek and the forehead. Directly afterwards, the patient spent 2 h in the hospital garden on a sunny day. After 2 h, the remaining MAL was washed off and physical sunscreen was applied to all of the face (fig. 5: left cheek immediately after the MAL-dPDT treatment). The patient reported only minor discomfort during this treatment with a mild burning sensation. He then left our outpatient clinic and was instructed to go home immediately and spend the rest of the day inside in order to avoid further activation of protoporphyrin IX.

Sixteen days after the first ingenol mebutate treatment and hence 6 days after the MAL-dPDT treatment, we saw the patient again. Erythema had returned to normal levels on both sides. We observed comparable efficacy in the treatment of thin actinic keratoses (fig. 6: right cheek, 16 days after the beginning of a 3 day course of ingenol mebutate 150 µg/g gel; fig. 7: left cheek, 6 days after MAL-dPDT treatment). Please note that thicker plaques and ulcerations were unchanged by treatment. These are beyond the indications for either field treatment used and were thus excised afterward.

We present this case in order to demonstrate feasibility, document patient discomfort and clinical outcome of ingenol mebutate in comparison with MAL-dPDT. Treatment with ingenol mebutate does not necessitate any preparation before the application or any special care afterwards. The process of application is completed in about 30 s per day. If the patient is able to apply a cream to the site of the treatment, he/she will be able to perform the therapy by him/herself. If necessary, limits can be drawn with a pen in order to identify the area of treatment, as was the case in our patient. We recommend covering the zone of application by a simple dressing in order to reduce brushing against the zone and – in case of a facial lesion – to improve social appearance. It is imperative to explain the process of desired reactions including pustules and crusts, redness and oozing prior to the treatment. Colour tables provided by the manufacturer of the gel can be helpful. Our patient reported only minor discomfort after the treatment due to a mild burning sensation. Ten days after the first application, we saw only mild irritation left. We achieved complete clearance of actinic keratoses without discoloration of the skin 16 days after ingenol mebutate 150 μg/g gel therapy. This treatment is officially registered for a surface of up to 25 cm^2 at a time [3].

For MAL-dPDT, preparation before the treatment (sunscreen, curettage) and special care after the treatment (washing the face, sunscreen, avoidance of further exposition to visible light) are necessary. This can, however, be done in one day. Post-treatment redness, crusting, pustules and oozing are similar to the ingenol mebutate treatment and must be addressed explicitly before the treatment. Our patient reported only mild discomfort due to a mild burning sensation. This is typical for the treatment and is generally well tolerated. We achieved complete clearance of thin actinic keratoses after 6 days, when irritation had returned to baseline.

MAL-dPDT treatment was a feasible, repeatable, physician-directed method of treating field cancerization with a limited down-time of around 6 days. Treatment with ingenol mebutate gel was a feasible, repeatable, physician-directed method of treating field cancerization with a down-time of around 10 days in this immunosuppressed patient. We expect this patient to undergo numerous treatments in the future as a consequence of his immunosuppression. He will be able to apply the ingenol mebutate treatment himself on the next occasion. At the time of treatment, the MAL-dPDT ran at 3 times the cost of ingenol mebutate gel.

Acknowledgments

The author would like to thank Dr. Evangelia Tzika (ingenol mebutate) and Dr. Donato Ferrara (MAL-dPDT) who were in charge of the treatments at the Division of Dermatology and Venereology, Geneva University Hospitals, Switzerland.

Statement of Ethics

The patient gave informed consent prior to the treatments.

Disclosure Statement

The author has previously received financial support for lectures and travel from LEO Pharma and Galderma Schweiz AG. Neither company was involved in the process of this article.

References

1 Werner RN, Stockfleth E, Connolly SM, Correia O, Erdmann R, Foley P, Gupta AK, Jacobs A, Kerl H, Lim HW, Martin G, Paquet M, Pariser DM, Rosumeck S, Röwert-Huber HJ, Sahota A, Sangueza OP, Shumack S, Sporbeck B, Swanson NA, Torezan L, Nast A: Evidence- and consensus-based (S3) guidelines for the treatment of actinic keratosis – international league of dermatological societies in cooperation with the European dermatology forum – short version. J Eur Acad Dermatol Venereol 2015;29: 2069–2079.

2 Hofbauer G, Anliker M, Boehncke WH, Brand C, Braun R, Gaide O, Hafner J, Hunger R, Itin P, Kaeuper G, Lautenschlager S, Mainetti C, Streit M: Swiss clinical practice guidelines on field cancerization of the skin. Swiss Med Wkly 2014;144:w14026.

3 Fachinformation: Picato® 150 mcg/g, Gel, Picato® 500 mcg/g, Gel. http://www.swissmedicinfo.ch/ShowText.aspx?textType=FI&lang=DE&authNr=62763.

4 Gaide O, Hofbauer G, Hunger R, Mühlstädt M, Plaza T: Consensus on daylight photodynamic therapy (dl-PDT) in Switzerland. Derm Hel 2015;27:34–37.

Dermatology

Dermatology 2016;232(suppl 1):24–28
DOI: 10.1159/000447393

Published online: August 11, 2016

Ingenol Mebutate for Lentigo Maligna: A Case Report

Karolina Gadaldi Laurence Feldmeyer Nikhil Yawalkar Robert E. Hunger

Department of Dermatology, University Hospital Inselspital, University of Bern, Bern, Switzerland

Key Words
Ingenol mebutate · Lentigo maligna · Melanoma · Treatment

Abstract
Background: Lentigo maligna (LM) is a melanoma in situ on sun-damaged skin, with a strong predilection to the head and neck area of the elderly. Many therapeutic modalities have been proposed in the treatment of this pathology, including surgery, cryotherapy, radiotherapy and topical imiquimod. Up to date surgical excision remains the treatment of choice with the lowest recurrence rate. Recently, a new topical treatment with ingenol mebutate has been described to be efficacious and well tolerated in the treatment of melanoma in situ. ***Objective:*** We sought to demonstrate that ingenol mebutate might be an efficacious and well-tolerated treatment in a patient suffering from LM on an aesthetically challenging location. ***Methods:*** Case report. ***Results:*** After therapeutic failure with imiquimod 5% cream, a new topical treatment with ingenol mebutate gel 0.015% once daily on 3 consecutive days was initiated. Despite visible inflammation, no macroscopic lesion clearance was observed. While the first follow-up using reflectance confocal microscopy (RCM) performed at 6 weeks after the completion of the therapy showed no signs of LM, the second follow-up examination at 12 weeks using RCM and biopsy confirmed recurrence of the lesion. ***Conclusion:*** Ingenol mebutate cannot be considered a standard treatment modality for all types of LM. Further studies are needed to evaluate the prerequisites that can ensure therapeutic success.

© 2016 S. Karger AG, Basel

Introduction

Lentigo maligna (LM) is a melanoma in situ of chronically sun-exposed skin, particularly, of the head and neck area [1]. It develops mainly in elderly patients. When untreated, LM is associated with a 5–50% risk of progressing to invasive LM melanoma, but the exact determinants for this transformation are still to be elucidated [2, 3]. Many therapeutic modalities, including surgery, cryotherapy, radiotherapy and imiquimod cream, have demonstrated an efficacy in the treatment of LM [4]. Surgical excision employing safety margins (usually micrographically controlled) remains the first-line therapy for this pathology. Recently, a new topical treatment with ingenol mebutate (0.015% gel) has been described to be efficacious and well tolerated in the treatment of melanoma in situ [5].

We present a case of a patient with LM on the face who was treated with ingenol mebutate, but relapsed 3 months after treatment.

KARGER

E-Mail karger@karger.com
www.karger.com/drm

© 2016 S. Karger AG, Basel
1018–8665/16/2327–0024$39.50/0

Dr. Karolina Gadaldi
Department of Dermatology
University Hospital Inselspital, University of Berne
CH–3010 Bern (Switzerland)
E-Mail karolina.gadaldi@insel.ch

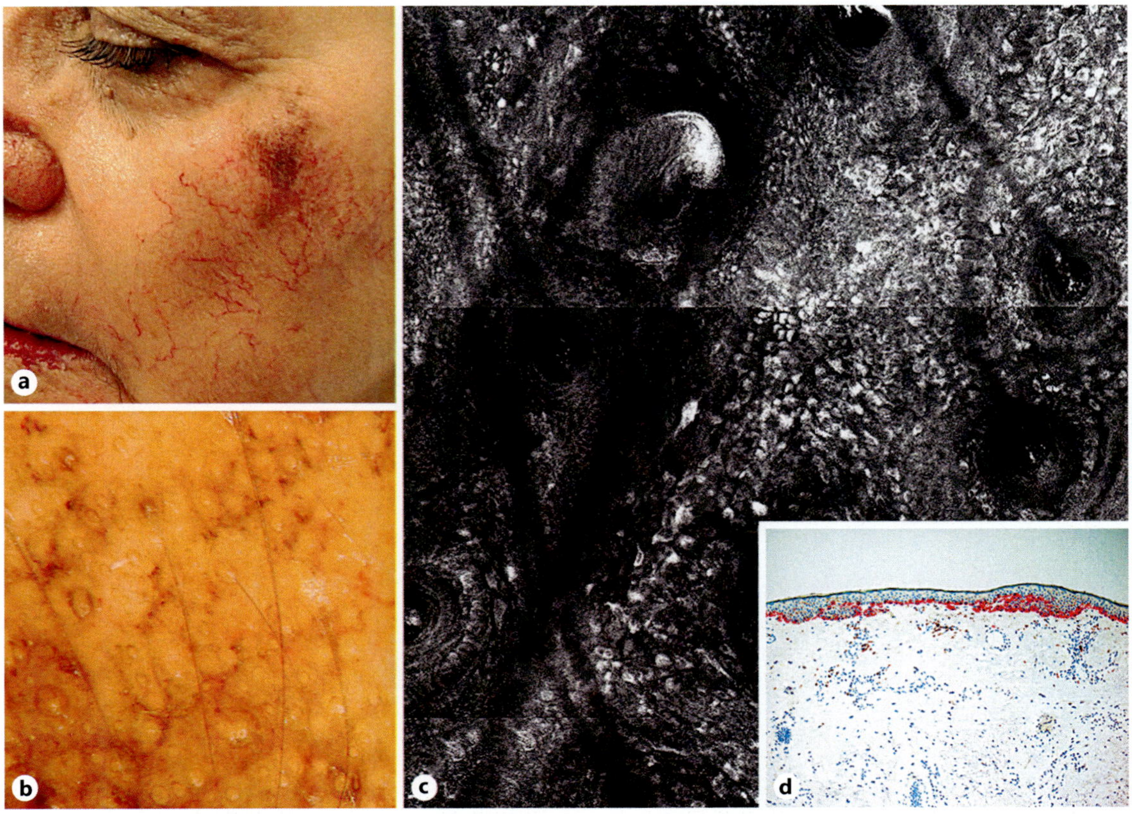

Fig. 1. Clinical (**a**), dermoscopic (**b**), confocal (**c**) and histological (**d**) picture of LM at baseline.

Case Report

A 70-year-old Caucasian woman, with a history of a multifocal hepatocellular carcinoma with pulmonary and lymph node metastases, presented to our outpatient clinic with a pigmented and slowly, but gradually enlarging macule on the face. The physical examination including dermoscopy showed a poorly demarcated light to dark brown macule measuring 2 × 1 cm with black dots and asymmetric pigmented follicular openings on her left cheekbone. The lesion was further examined by reflectance confocal microscopy (RCM; Vivascope 1500, Mavig AG, Germany) revealing a disturbed architecture of the epidermis with a presence of numerous, large, round and dendritic pleomorphic cells, distributed in all epidermal layers, suggesting pagetoid spread of atypical melanocytes. An increased proliferation of atypical melanocytes was observed especially along adnexal structures. In the dermis, non-edged papillae and solar damage were the commonest findings (fig. 1). Histological examination of the 4-mm punch biopsy specimen taken in the area guided by RCM confirmed the diagnosis of LM (fig. 1).

Informed consent for image acquisition, biopsy specimen sampling and treatment (including evidence-based and off-label use) was obtained from the patient. On account of her age and comorbidities, as well as the cosmetically challenging localization and size of the lesion, the patient declined a surgery.

Therefore, an alternative treatment with imiquimod cream 5% was initiated. The patient was instructed to apply the cream, covering the affected area and a 1-cm margin of the surrounding skin twice daily 7 days a week. After 8 weeks of treatment, no inflammatory reaction was observed. Hence, the topical treatment was changed to ingenol mebutate gel 0.015%. Three consecutive daily applications of the gel were performed on the lesion and 1 cm of the adjacent skin once daily for 3 days. At the end of the 3-day treatment a strong inflammatory, crusting and oozing reaction on the application site developed (fig. 2).

In the follow-up RCM examination, at 6 weeks after completion of the treatment, no criteria for LM were found. Clinically and dermoscopically, a lentiginous pigmented macule was still visible on the face (fig. 3). The follow-up examination with RCM performed after 12 weeks of treatment with ingenol mebutate showed a relapse of the LM. A 4-mm punch biopsy confirmed LM (fig. 4).

Discussion

Ingenol mebutate is a hydrophobic diterpene ester isolated from a sap of a plant *Euphorbia peplus*, commonly known as a 'petty spurge' in the United Kingdom or 'radium weed' in Australia, that has a long tradition of use for a variety of conditions, including skin cancer [6]. Ingenol mebutate has been registered in the USA

Dermatology 2016;232(suppl 1):24–28
DOI: 10.1159/000447393

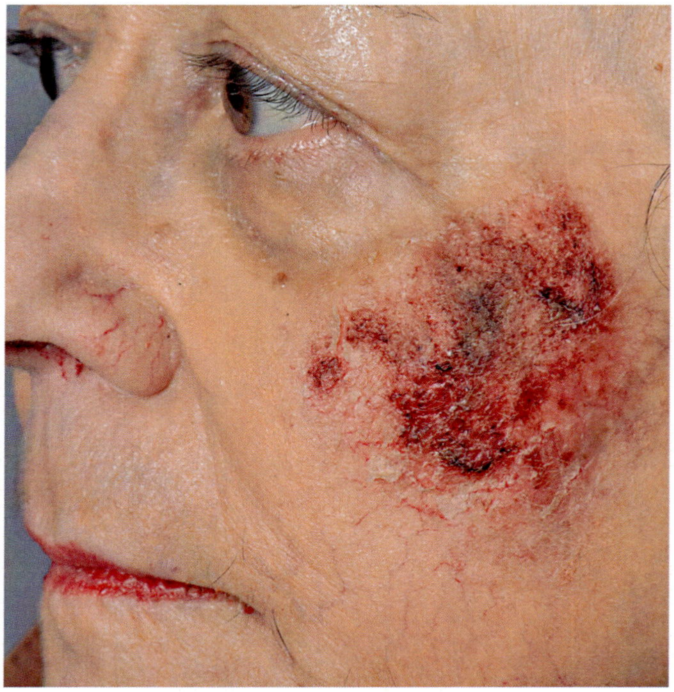

Fig. 2. Strong local inflammatory response after the treatment with ingenol mebutate.

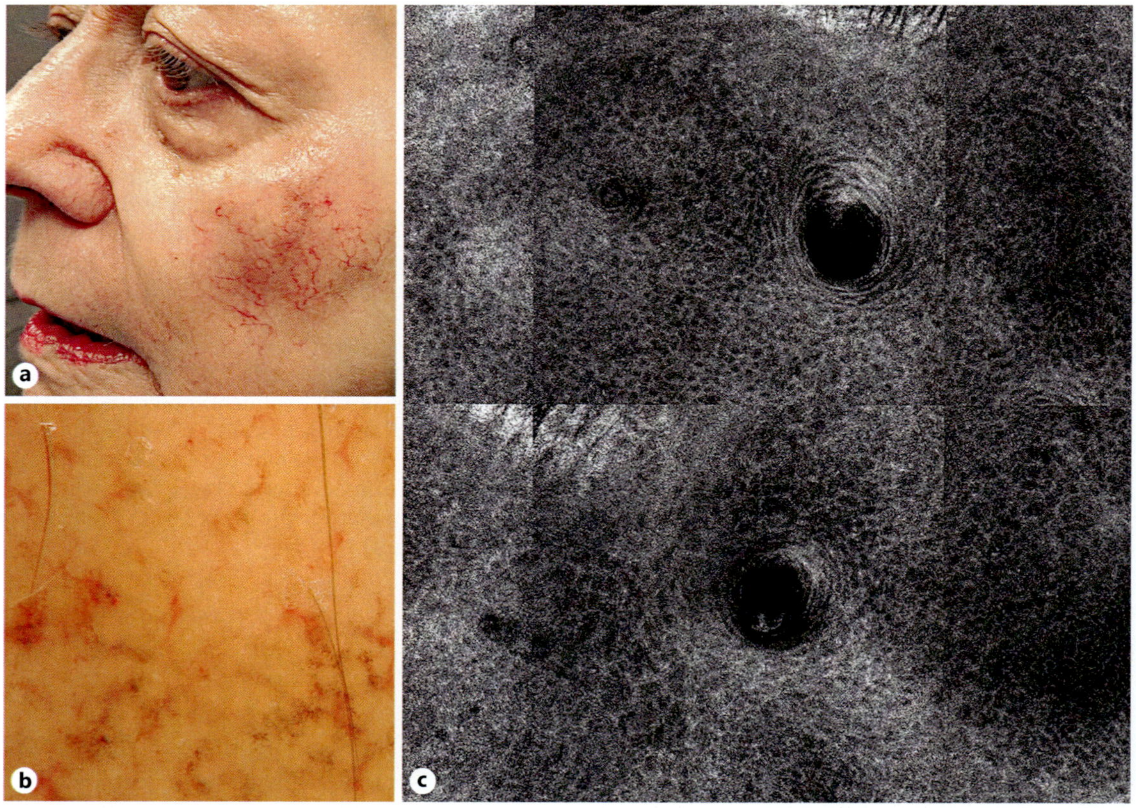

Fig. 3. Clinical (**a**), dermoscopic (**b**) and confocal picture (**c**) of LM at 6 weeks after the treatment with ingenol mebutate.

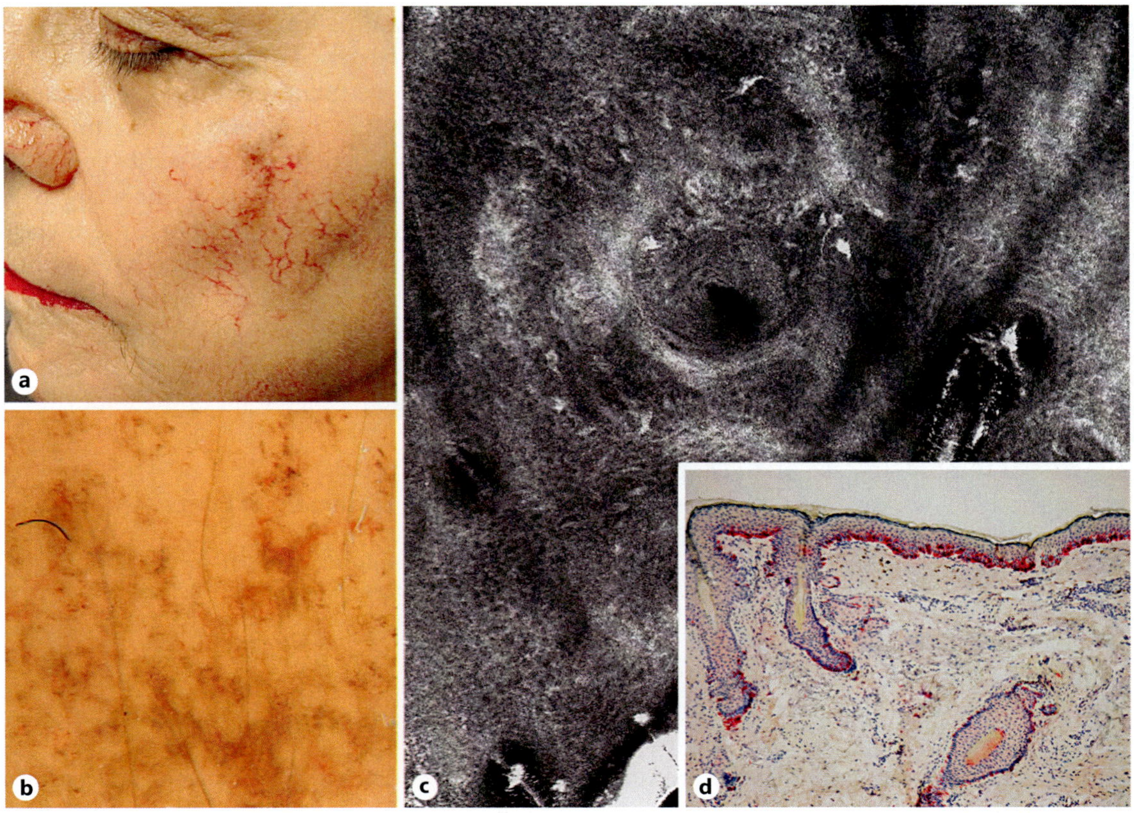

Fig. 4. Clinical (**a**), dermoscopic (**b**), confocal (**c**) and histological (**d**) picture of a recurrent LM at 12 weeks after the treatment with ingenol mebutate.

and Europa as a local treatment for actinic keratosis [7–10]. In addition to its approved use, ingenol mebutate has emerged in the last years as an efficient topical agent for the treatment of Bowen's disease [11], superficial basal cell carcinoma [12] and molluscum contagiosum [13].

To date, there is only one report on successful treatment of recurrent melanoma in situ with ingenol mebutate (0.015% for 3 days) at 6 months of follow-up [5].

Ingenol mebutate has been demonstrated to induce both non-apoptotic and apoptotic cell death in several malignant cell lines, including melanoma. Analysis of murine melanoma cells in vivo and in vitro with an electron microscopy confirmed a relatively rapid necrotic cell death after disintegration of the plasma membrane and disruption of cytoplasmic organelles with a loss of mitochondrial potential, following an exposure to topical ingenol mebutate [14]. The same study demonstrated a necrosis of other tumor cell lines (including human prostate carcinoma, breast adenocarcinoma and acute leukemia) confirming cytotoxic cell death and consequently low specificity of the drug at the concentrations used for different tumor cell types. Development of a rapid, strong, cytotoxic reaction as described above was also observed in our case.

Apart from its cytotoxic properties, ingenol mebutate is a protein kinase C activator [15] and induces apoptosis in caspase-dependent way [16]. In an in vitro study on different melanoma cell lines, ingenol mebutate induced cell death in all of the cultured melanoma cell lines. However, only in 20% of human melanoma cell lines was cell death a result of apoptosis, the rest resulting from necrosis. The exact mechanism of melanoma cell lines sensitivity to apoptosis after treatment with ingenol mebutate has not been completely elucidated.

Cozzi et al. [17] observed that treatment with ingenol mebutate caused a selective and irreversible induction of cell senescence in only certain sensitive melanoma cell lines. *BRAF* genotypes of the melanoma cell lines used in the study showed no correlation with the treatment outcome, with all sensitive cell lines mutated at either *NRAS* or *BRAF* loci. The authors hypothesize that the induction of senescence in some of the melanoma cell lines might have been achieved by activation of MAPK pathway. Moreover, the tumor suppressor gene *HRASL3/*

Dermatology 2016;232(suppl 1):24–28
DOI: 10.1159/000447393

HREV107 was higher expressed in melanoma cell lines resistant to ingenol mebutate treatment. Hence, they speculate that certain criteria must be present to render melanoma cells susceptible to senescence, namely, the presence of an activating *NRAS* or *BRAF* mutation and low transcriptional levels of the MAPK inhibitor *HREV107*.

In our patient, treatment of LM with ingenol mebutate led to a transient clearance of melanoma cells, confirmed by RCM examination, but did not result in remission of the lesion.

The described therapeutic effect of ingenol mebutate is superficial and is therefore expected to act mainly in superficial tumors. In case of a LM, proliferating melanocytes may penetrate deep into the skin, along the adnexal structures. Hence, the reduced absorption/penetration of the drug might explain the therapeutic failure. RCM is a non-invasive imaging technique that enables in vivo visualization of the epidermis down to the papillary dermis in real time. Resolution is almost comparable to conventional histology. Therefore, incompletely eliminated melanoma cells from the lower levels of the hair follicle's isthmus might have been undetectable on examination. Rapid recurrence of the lesion suggests the persistence of melanoma cells. Moreover, based on the above-mentioned in vitro studies, we can hypothesize that the therapeutic failure might have been caused also by a genetically resistant type of melanoma cells or by insufficient dose of the drug needed for a complete clearance. Furthermore, the metastasizing hepatocellular carcinoma may also have hampered the immune reaction against the melanoma cells. Further studies, especially in vivo and on larger series of subjects are needed to better evaluate the efficacy of the treatment with ingenol mebutate in melanocytic tumors.

Statement of Ethics

Informed consent for image acquisition, biopsy specimen sampling and treatment (including evidence-based and off-label use) was obtained from the patient.

Disclosure Statement

The authors declare no conflict of interest.

References

1 Ciocan D, Barbe C, Aubin F, Granel-Brocard F, Lipsker D, Velten M, Dalac S, Truchetet F, Michel C, Mitschler A, Arnoult G, Buemi A, Dalle S, Bernard P, Woronoff AS, Grange F: Distinctive features of melanoma and its management in elderly patients: a population-based study in France. JAMA Dermatol 2013;149:1150–1157.

2 Tannous ZS, Lerner LH, Duncan LM, Mihm MC Jr, Flotte TJ: Progression to invasive melanoma from malignant melanoma in situ, lentigo maligna type. Hum Pathol 2000;31:705–708.

3 Erickson C, Miller SJ: Treatment options in melanoma in situ: topical and radiation therapy, excision and Mohs surgery. Int J Dermatol 2010;49:482–491.

4 Higgins HW 2nd, Lee KC, Galan A, Leffell DJ: Melanoma in situ: part II. Histopathology, treatment, and clinical management. J Am Acad Dermatol 2015;73:193–203; quiz 203–204.

5 Mansuy M, Nikkels-Tassoudji N, Arrese JE, Rorive A, Nikkels AF: Recurrent in situ melanoma successfully treated with ingenol mebutate. Dermatol Ther (Heidelb) 2014;4:131–135.

6 Ramsay JR, Suhrbier A, Aylward JH, Ogbourne S, Cozzi SJ, Poulsen MG, Baumann KC, Welburn P, Redlich GL, Parsons PG: The sap from Euphorbia peplus is effective against human nonmelanoma skin cancers. Br J Dermatol 2011;164:633–636.

7 Lebwohl M, Shumack S, Stein Gold L, Melgaard A, Larsson T, Tyring SK: Long-term follow-up study of ingenol mebutate gel for the treatment of actinic keratoses. JAMA Dermatol 2013;149:666–670.

8 Keating GM: Ingenol mebutate gel 0.015% and 0.05%: in actinic keratosis. Drugs 2012;72:2397–2405.

9 Ottawa (ON): Canadian Agency for Drugs and Technologies in Health: Ingenol Mebutate (Picato): Topical Treatment of Non-Hyperkeratotic, Non-Hypertrophic Actinic Keratosis in Adults. CADTH Common Drug Reviews, 2014.

10 Anderson L, Schmieder GJ, Werschler WP, Tschen EH, Ling MR, Stough DB, Katsamas J: Randomized, double-blind, double-dummy, vehicle-controlled study of ingenol mebutate gel 0.025% and 0.05% for actinic keratosis. J Am Acad Dermatol 2009;60:934–943.

11 Braun SA, Homey B, Gerber PA: [Successful treatment of Bowen disease with ingenol mebutate]. Hautarzt 2014;65:848–850.

12 Cantisani C, Paolino G, Cantoresi F, Faina V, Richetta AG, Calvieri S: Superficial basal cell carcinoma successfully treated with ingenol mebutate gel 0.05%. Dermatol Ther 2014;27:352–354.

13 Javed S, Tyring SK: Treatment of molluscum contagiosum with ingenol mebutate. J Am Acad Dermatol 2014;70:e105.

14 Ogbourne SM, Suhrbier A, Jones B, Cozzi SJ, Boyle GM, Morris M, McAlpine D, Johns J, Scott TM, Sutherland KP, Gardner JM, Le TT, Lenarczyk A, Aylward JH, Parsons PG: Antitumor activity of 3-ingenyl angelate: plasma membrane and mitochondrial disruption and necrotic cell death. Cancer Res 2004;64:2833–2839.

15 Ersvaer E, Kittang AO, Hampson P, Sand K, Gjertsen BT, Lord JM, Bruserud O: The protein kinase C agonist PEP005 (ingenol 3-angelate) in the treatment of human cancer: a balance between efficacy and toxicity. Toxins (Basel) 2010;2:174–194.

16 Gillespie SK, Zhang XD, Hersey P: Ingenol 3-angelate induces dual modes of cell death and differentially regulates tumor necrosis factor-related apoptosis-inducing ligand-induced apoptosis in melanoma cells. Mol Cancer Ther 2004;3:1651–1658.

17 Cozzi SJ, Parsons PG, Ogbourne SM, Pedley J, Boyle GM: Induction of senescence in diterpene ester-treated melanoma cells via protein kinase C-dependent hyperactivation of the mitogen-activated protein kinase pathway. Cancer Res 2006;66:10083–10091.

Dermatology

Dermatology 2016;232(suppl 1):29–31
DOI: 10.1159/000447394

Published online: August 11, 2016

Ingenol Mebutate Treatment in a Patient with Gorlin Syndrome

Marco Stieger Robert E. Hunger

Department of Dermatology, University Hospital Inselspital, University of Bern, Bern, Switzerland

Key Words
Gorlin syndrome · Basal cell nevus syndrome · Ingenol mebutate · Basal cell carcinoma · PTCH1 gene mutation · Vismodegib

Abstract
Background: Gorlin syndrome, also known as the basal cell nevus syndrome (OMIM #109400), is a rare autosomal-dominant genetic disease. The disease, which shows mutation of the patched receptor gene (*PTCH1*) of the sonic hedgehog pathway, is characterized by developing multiple basal cell carcinomas (BCCs) in adolescent patients. Other clinical features include mandibular keratocysts, palmar and plantar pits, skeletal abnormalities and malformations central nervous system and genital tract. Gorlin–Goltz patients need multidisciplinary medical care and follow-up as well as genetic counseling if the patients want to have children. The treatment of multiple BCCs includes conventional surgery, micrographic Mohs surgery, cryotherapy, laser ablation, photodynamic therapy, imiquimod 5% cream, 5-fluorouracil cream as well as the sonic hedgehog pathway inhibitor vismodegib. ***Case Report:*** We report the case of a 30-year-old woman seen in our dermatological department since 2003. All the above-mentioned modalities had been employed for her numerous BCCs. The patient grew wary of the surgical procedures because of the countless scars. We successfully treated multiple BCCs with ingenol mebutate without post-inflammatory scarring. At 8-month follow-up, the patient shows no recurrence of the treated lesions. ***Conclusion:*** Ingenol mebutate can be used to treat (superficial) BCCs in patients with Gorlin–Goltz syndrome as an additional modality. Close clinical follow-up is recommended.

© 2016 S. Karger AG, Basel

Introduction

Gorlin syndrome, also known as the basal cell nevus syndrome (OMIM #109400), is a rare autosomal-dominant genetic disease. The characteristic multiorgan abnormalities are caused by mutations of the patched receptor gene (*PTCH1*), a tumor suppressor gene, on chromosome arm 9q. *PTCH1* inhibits signaling by the membrane protein Smoothened (SMO). The loss-of-function mutation of *PCHT1* results in an elevated activation of the sonic hedgehog pathway, which activates transcription factors such as GLI1. GLI1 induces cell cycle progression and cell proliferation and is associated in development of basal cell carcinoma (BCC) and medulloblastoma. Up to 40% of the patients show a de-novo mutation with negative family history. The prevalence is 1:60,000 with an equal frequency in women and men [1, 2].

Most patients develop multiple BCCs already in adolescence, which should raise the suspicion of Gorlin–Goltz syndrome. The BCCs are usually located on the face and trunk, but also occur on sun-protected areas. All histological subtypes from superficial to infiltrative and morphoeic BCC can be found. Aggressive forms such as the locally destroying ulcus terebrans are very rare. Other

KARGER

E-Mail karger@karger.com
www.karger.com/drm

© 2016 S. Karger AG, Basel
1018–8665/16/2327–0029$39.50/0

Marco Stieger
Department of Dermatology
University Hospital Inselspital, University of Bern
CH–3010 Bern (Switzerland)
E-Mail marco.stieger@insel.ch

1

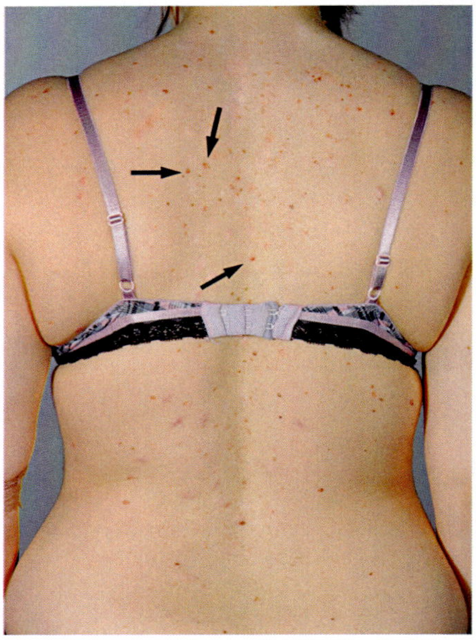

2

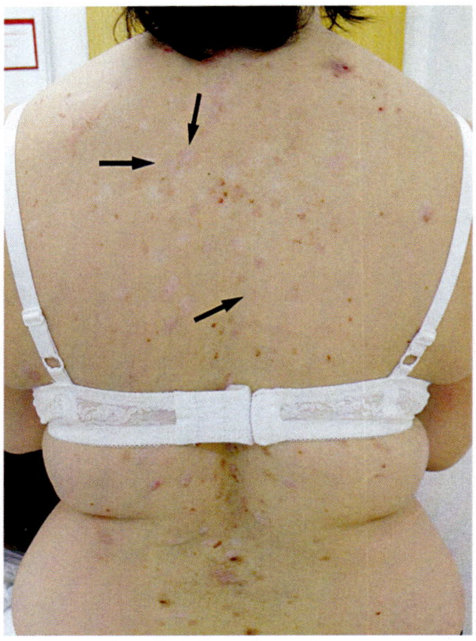

Fig. 1. Multiple clinically diagnosed BCC (arrows).

Fig. 2. Complete resolution of the BCC after topical treatment with ingenol mebutate gel (arrows).

clinical features include mandibular keratocysts, palmar and plantar pits, skeletal abnormalities and malformations in the central nervous system and genital tract. Gorlin–Goltz patients need multidisciplinary medical care and follow-up as well as genetic counseling if the patients want to have children [3].

The treatment of multiple BCCs includes conventional surgery, micrographic Mohs surgery, cryotherapy, laser ablation, curettage and electrodessication, photodynamic therapy, imiquimod 5% cream, 5-fluorouracil cream as well as the sonic hedgehog pathway inhibitor vismodegib. Radiotherapy is contraindicated, since further BCCs could be induced, where the mutation of the *PTCH1* gene causes an increased sensitivity to radiation [4, 5].

Ingenol mebutate is approved as a topical treatment of actinic keratosis. It is believed that the local effect inhibits the growth of cancer cells and/or induces tumor cell death. The incidence of local skin reactions is high, and it has proven to be safe and efficacious. Successful off-label treatment of superficial BCCs with ingenol mebutate has previously been shown [6].

Case Report

A 30-year-old Caucasian woman was diagnosed with Gorlin–Goltz syndrome in 2003, when multiple BCCs were detected. The diagnosis was based on clinical features such as palmar pits, hypertelorism, increased head circumference, calcification of the falx cerebri, multiple ovarian cysts and fibromas and the radiologic evidence of odontogenic keratocysts. Genotyping of the *PTCH1* gene detected a heterozygous mutation. Over 10 years, the patient was treated with numerous procedures such as micrographic Mohs surgery, conventional surgery, photodynamic therapy and topical therapy with imiquimod cream. In 2014, we initiated a systemic therapy with vismodegib, which showed a pronounced response with decrease of most of the BCC. The patient developed alopecia, dysgeusia and pronounced long-lasting fatigue. Eventually, the patient decided to stop vismodegib therapy after 6 months on account of side effects impairing her quality of life. BCC recurred after 3 months but the patient was tired of surgery and asked for an alternative therapy. Cryosurgery was very painful and also resulted in extensive scarring. We treated multiple BCCs on her back with 500 μg/g of ingenol mebutate gel (fig. 1). Her husband applied the gel for 2 consecutive days. She reported a local inflammatory reaction, which healed after 2 weeks. Clinically, the treated BCCs showed complete resolution without scarring (fig. 2). The patient repeated the treatment on a regular basis without affecting her daily life and work. During the follow-up over 8 months, no recurrence of the treated BCC was detected. Of course, occasional surgery of more invasive BCCs was not completely unavoidable but the patient was happy to be able to treat many BCCs on her own without a great effort and side effects.

Conclusion

Ingenol mebutate seems a suitable off-label option to treat (superficial) BCCs in patients with Gorlin syndrome. The treatment is easy to manage and patients appreciate being able to treat autonomously.

Statement of Ethics

Informed consent for image acquisition, biopsy specimen sampling and treatment (including evidence-based and off-label use) was obtained from the patient.

Disclosure Statement

The authors declare no conflicts of interest.

References

1 Bonifas JM, Pennypacker S, Chuang PT, et al: Activation of expression of hedgehog target genes in basal cell carcinomas. J Invest Dermatol 2001;116:739–742.
2 Pino LC, Balassiano LK, et al: Basal cell nevus syndrome: clinical and molecular review and case report. Int J Dermatol 2016;55:367–375.
3 Acocella A, Sacco R, Bertolai R, Sacco N: Genetic and clinicopathologic aspects of Gorlin-Goltz syndrome (NBCCS): presentation of two case reports and literature review. Minerva Stomatol 2009;58:43–53.
4 Baliga SD, Rao SS: Nevoid-basal cell carcinoma syndrome: a case report and overview on diagnosis and management. J Maxillofac Oral Surg 2010;9:82–86.
5 Weiss GJ, Tibes R, et al: Long-term safety, tolerability, and efficacy of vismodegib in two patients with metastatic basal cell carcinoma and basal cell nevus syndrome. Dermatol Reports 2011;3:e55.
6 Cantisani C, Paolino G, et al: Superficial basal cell carcinoma successfully treated with ingenol mebutate gel 0.05%. Dermatol Ther 2014;27:352–354.

Dermatology

Author Index Vol. 232, Suppl 1, 2016

Subject Index Vol. 232, Suppl 1, 2016

© 2016 S. Karger AG, Basel

E-Mail karger@karger.com
www.karger.com/drm

Concise insights into a beneficial therapy

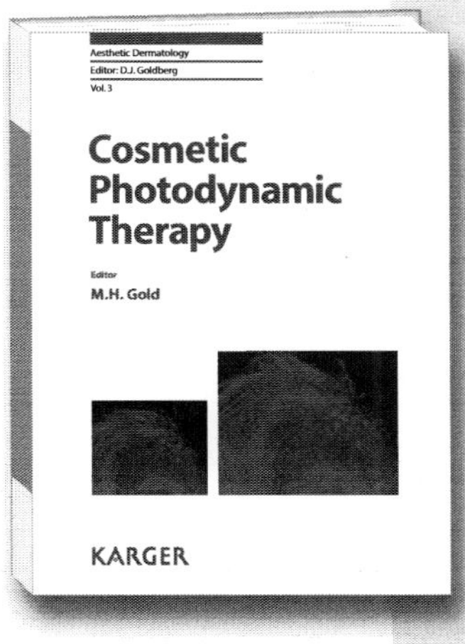

Cosmetic Photodynamic Therapy

Editor
Michael H. Gold

Cosmetic Photodynamic Therapy
Editor: Gold, M.H. (Nashville, Tenn.)
VIII + 136 p., 34 fig., 26 in color, 10 tab., 2016
CHF 112.00 / EUR 105.00 / USD 132.00
(hard cover)
CHF 134.00 / EUR 126.00 / USD 158.00 (online)
Online version for institutional purchase
Prices subject to change, VAT not included
EUR price for eurozone countries, USD price for USA and Latin America only
ISBN 978-3-318-02556-9 (hard cover)
e-ISBN 978-3-318-02557-6

Aesthetic Dermatology, Vol. 3
Series Editor: Goldberg, D.J. (New York, N.Y.)

Photodynamic Therapy (PDT) has become an important treatment modality in medical practice. New and exciting applications continue to emerge and the future of PDT looks brighter and brighter. Dermatologists and other health professionals around the world rely on its therapeutic effect for the treatment of actinic keratoses, non-melanoma skin cancers, acne vulgaris, and various other dermatologic conditions.
In this comprehensive yet concise book, world-renowned experts showcase all of the common, everyday uses of PDT in dermatologic offices. They also examine how this beneficial therapy can be utilized to its full capacity. The considerable knowledge presented here renders this publication an indispensable resource for all dermatologists and health professionals who offer their patients this effective, noninvasive procedure.

Contents

Dear Librarian

I have reviewed this publication and would like to recommend it for our library.

Recommended by:

Department:

Date:

Signature:

Orders may be placed with any bookshop, subscription agency, directly with the publisher or through a Karger distributor.

The easiest way to order: **www.karger.com/aesde**

Karger – Medical and Scientific Publishers
CH–4009 Basel, Switzerland
orders@karger.com, f: +41 61 306 12 34
www.karger.com

KI16214

KARGER

The venue for research on new drugs and therapeutic concepts

Skin Pharmacology and Physiology

Journal of Pharmacological and Biophysical Research

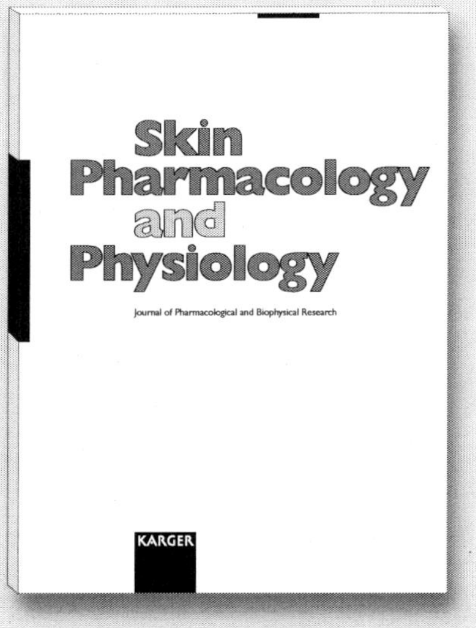

Editor
J. Lademann, Berlin

Honorary Editor
H.F. Merk, Aachen

Associate Editors
P. Elias, San Francisco, Calif.
J.W. Fluhr, Berlin
H.I. Maibach, San Francisco, Calif.
H. Mukhtar, Madison, Wis.
G. Nohynek, Asnières
M. Roberts, Brisbane, Qld.
C. Surber, Basel
P. van de Kerkhof, Nijmegen

Official Organ of the
Society for Dermopharmacy

In the past decade research into skin pharmacology has rapidly developed with new and promising drugs and therapeutic concepts being introduced regularly. Recently, the use of nanoparticles for drug delivery in dermatology and cosmetology has become a topic of intensive research, yielding remarkable and in part surprising results. Another topic of current research is the use of tissue tolerable plasma in wound treatment. Stimulating not only wound healing processes but also the penetration of topically applied substances into the skin, this novel technique is expected to deliver very interesting results.
There are many open questions which reflect the importance of the subject and the need for an international scientific forum where they can be discussed in extenso. Dermatologists, pharmaceutical chemists, pharmacologists, toxicologists, and others interested in the subject are invited to contribute and to submit their best research work for publication in *Skin Pharmacology and Physiology.*

Skin Pharmacology and Physiology
Founded: 1988
Category: Clinical and Basic Research
Fields of Interest: Pharmacology, Dermatology

Listed in bibliographic services, including *Journal Citation Reports, PubMed/MEDLINE, Biological Abstracts, Embase, KOSMET*

2016: Volume 29
6 issues per volume
Language: English
ISSN 1660–5527
e-ISSN 1660–5535

Impact Factor: 2.366

Selected contributions

- The Antimicrobial Peptides Psoriasin (S100A7) and Koebnerisin (S100A15) Suppress Extracellular Matrix Production and Proliferation of Human Fibroblasts: **Gauglitz, G.G.; Bureik, D.; Zwicker, S.; Ruzicka, T.; Wolf, R.** (Munich)
- pH Influence on Antibacterial Efficacy of Common Antiseptic Substances: **Wiegand, C.** (Jena); **Abel, M.** (Rengsdorf); **Ruth, P.** (Neuwied); **Elsner, P.; Hipler, U.-C.** (Jena)
- Metrics and Clinical Relevance of Percutaneous Penetration and Lateral Spreading: **Vieille-Petit, A.** (San Francisco, Calif./Lyon); **Blickenstaff, N.; Coman, G.; Maibach, H.** (San Francisco, Calif.)
- Novel in vitro Approaches for the Simulation and Analysis of Human Skin Wounds: **Planz, V.; Franzen, L.; Windbergs, M.** (Saarbruecken)
- What Is Sensitive Skin? A Systematic Literature Review of Objective Measurements: **Richters, R.; Falcone, D.** (Nijmegen); **Uzunbajakava, N.; Verkruysse, W.** (Eindhoven); **van Erp, P.; van de Kerkhof, P.** (Nijmegen)
- An in vitro Skin Penetration Model for Compromised Skin: Estimating Penetration of Polyethylene Glycol [^{14}C]-PEG-7 Phosphate: **Dey, S.** (Cincinnati, Ohio); **Rothe, H.** (Darmstadt); **Page, L.** (Tranent); **O'Connor, R.; Farahmand, S.** (Cincinnati, Ohio); **Toner, F.** (Tranent); **Marsh, R.; Wehmeyer, K.; Zhou, S.** (Cincinnati, Ohio)
- Porcine Ear Skin as a Biological Substrate for in vitro Testing of Sunscreen Performance: **Sohn, M.; Korn, V.** (Muttenz); **Imanidis, G.** (Muttenz/Basel)
- Skin Diseases Associated with the Depletion of Stratum Corneum Lipids and Stratum Corneum Lipid Substitution Therapy: **Sahle, F.F.** (Halle (Saale)/Addis Ababa); **Gebre-Mariam, T.** (Addis Ababa); **Dobner, B.; Wohlrab, J.; Neubert, R.H.H.** (Halle (Saale))

More information at **www.karger.com/spp**

KF16102

KARGER